Ciba Foundation
Study Group No. 37

# HYPERTROPHIC OBSTRUCTIVE
# CARDIOMYOPATHY

# HYPERTROPHIC OBSTRUCTIVE CARDIOMYOPATHY

Ciba Foundation
Study Group No. 37

Edited by
G. E. W. WOLSTENHOLME
and
MAEVE O'CONNOR

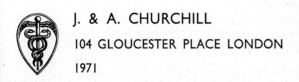

J. & A. CHURCHILL
104 GLOUCESTER PLACE LONDON
1971

First published 1971

With 86 illustrations

I.S.B.N. 0 7000 1509 4

*Printed in Great Britain*

4.3.71.

# Contents

# CONTENTS

# Membership

## Study Group on Hypertrophic Obstructive Cardiomyopathy held Friday 4th September 1970

**H. B. Burchell** . . Department of Medicine, Mayo Memorial
**(Chairman)** Building, University of Minnesota, Hospital
P.O. Box 94, Minneapolis, Minnesota 55455,
U.S.A.

**W. P. Cleland** . . Brompton Hospital, Institute of Diseases of the
**(Chairman)** Chest, Fulham Road, London S.W.3

**R. D. Teare** . . Department of Forensic Medicine, St George's
**(Chairman)** Hospital Medical School, Hyde Park Corner,
London, S.W.1

**B. G. Barratt-Boyes** . Cardiothoracic Surgical Unit, Green Lane
Hospital, Green Lane West, Auckland 3,
New Zealand

**H. H. Bentall** . . Department of Surgery, Royal Postgraduate
Medical School, Hammersmith Hospital,
Ducane Road, London, W.12

**E. Braunwald** . . Department of Medicine, University of California, University Hospital of San Diego County,
225 West Dickinson Street, San Diego,
California 92103, U.S.A.

**Lord Brock** . . Department of Surgical Sciences, Royal College
of Surgeons of England, 35–43 Lincoln's Inn
Fields, London, WC2A 3PN

**R. Emanuel** . . Department of Cardiology, The Middlesex
Hospital, London, W.1

**J. F. Goodwin** . . Department of Medicine, Royal Postgraduate
Medical School, Hammersmith Hospital,
Ducane Road, London, W.12

**Katherine A.**
**Hallidie-Smith** . Department of Medicine, Royal Postgraduate
Medical School, Hammersmith Hospital,
Ducane Road, London, W.12

**C. Grant** . . . Veterans Administration Hospital, Albany, New
York 12208, U.S.A.

**J. N. Homan**
**van der Heide** . . Department of Thoracic Surgery, University
Hospital, Oostersingel 59, Groningen, The
Netherlands

**A. Kristinsson** . . Medical Department, University Hospital, P.O. Box 1036, Reykjavik, Iceland

**I. S. Meerschwam** . Wilhelmina Gasthuis, Amsterdam, The Netherlands

**M. Nellen** . . . 903 Medical Centre, Heerengracht, Cape Town, South Africa

**Celia M. Oakley**. . Department of Medicine, Royal Postgraduate Medical School, Hammersmith Hospital, Ducane Road, London, W.12

**K. P. O'Brien** . . Auckland Hospital, Park Road, Auckland 3, New Zealand

**E. G. J. Olsen** . . Department of Pathology, Royal Postgraduate Medical School, Hammersmith Hospital, Ducane Road, London, W.12

**P. M. Shah** . . . School of Medicine and Dentistry, Strong Memorial Hospital, The University of Rochester, 260 Crittenden Boulevard, Rochester, New York 14620, U.S.A.

**M. D. Silver** . . Department of Pathology, Banting Institute, University of Toronto, 100 College Street, Toronto 2, Ontario, Canada

**Susan Van Noorden** . Department of Histochemistry, Royal Postgraduate Medical School, Hammersmith Hospital, Ducane Road, London, W.12

**M. M. Webb-Peploe** . Department of Medicine, Royal Postgraduate Medical School, Hammersmith Hospital, Ducane Road, London, W.12

**E. D. Wigle** . . Cardiovascular Unit, Toronto General Hospital, Toronto 2, Ontario, Canada

# The Ciba Foundation

The Ciba Foundation was opened in 1949 to promote international cooperation in medical and chemical research. It owes its existence to the generosity of CIBA Ltd (now CIBA-GEIGY Ltd), Basle, who, recognizing the obstacles to scientific communication created by war, man's natural secretiveness, disciplinary divisions, academic prejudices, distance, and differences of language, decided to set up a philanthropic institution whose aim would be to overcome such barriers. London was chosen as its site for reasons dictated by the special advantages of English charitable trust law (ensuring the independence of its actions), as well as those of language and geography.

The Foundation's house at 41 Portland Place, London, has become well known to workers in many fields of science. Every year the Foundation organizes six to ten three-day symposia and three or four shorter study groups, all of which are published in book form. Many other scientific meetings are held, organized either by the Foundation or by other groups in need of a meeting place. Accommodation is also provided for scientists visiting London, whether or not they are attending a meeting in the house.

The Foundation's many activities are controlled by a small group of distinguished trustees. Within the general framework of biological science, interpreted in its broadest sense, these activities are well summed up by the motto of the Ciba Foundation: *Consocient Gentes*—let the peoples come together.

# CHAIRMAN'S OPENING REMARKS

## Professor H. B. Burchell

First I wish to welcome the members of this study group. I do not know whether it is more fitting that special greetings be offered to those participants who were also present six years ago at the symposium on cardiomyopathies arranged by the Ciba Foundation (Wolstenholme and O'Connor 1964), or to those who come to this workshop unbiased and unencumbered by the presentations and active discussion of that meeting. Of the 23 persons listed to take part today, ten were participants in the earlier symposium (which I believe remains a standard reference on the topic of cardiomyopathy).

Sir John McMichael chaired that symposium in 1964 and in his opening remarks anticipated the spirit and the developments of the conference by stating "I have never before taken part in a discussion in which we start with so few fixed or preconceived ideas." He also gave a list of the names which had been coined to label 'cardiomyopathic syndromes' and stated ". . . . it may be part of our exercise in this discussion to clarify terminology." These insights may serve to point to the directions most profitable for discussion at this second conference; in particular, let us not start with rigid or fixed ideas. I am frankly disappointed that in 1964 I knew as much, in principle, about how the ventricle obstructs itself as I do now. I hope that at the end of this session I shall no longer be able to say this and can possibly admit to the rut which I have occupied.

May I direct your attention to some of the questions or problems which were asked or identified during the days of the first conference and which remain inadequately answered or solved:

(1) The nomenclature may still be confusing, particularly in respect of the variety of conditions which may present with 'idiopathic' ventricular hypertrophy.

(2) Does hypertrophy always precede the obstruction, or can the obstructive feature precede the hypertrophy? Is septal hypertrophy present before the general hypertrophy in the majority or the minority of the cases?

(3) Is the tiny end-systolic volume a constant finding and does active contraction always persist after completion of ejection?

(4) Have entrapment and obstruction, as factors in the left ventricular aortic pressure differences, been entirely clarified? How often do both occur?

(5) Is the site of the obstruction, namely between the septal bulge and anterior mitral leaflet, now agreed upon?

(6) How specific are the histological findings and what is their dynamic and aetiological significance?

(7) Is the ventricular excitation pattern abnormal, and specifically, is the hypothesis of early basilar contraction now discredited? What is the meaning of the short P-R interval, and the short P-R interval plus QRS aberration in some of the cases?

(8) How often do valvular aortic stenosis and essential hypertension precede hypertrophic obstruction and how often are they causally related to it?

(9) Are the genetic patterns established?

(10) What is the long-term prognosis, particularly in the members of family aggregates who are asymptomatic?

(11) What are the long-term results of surgical treatment?

(12) What are the long-term results of pharmacological (propranolol) treatment?

(13) Has true regression of the disease been observed?

(14) What is the relationship, if any, with the 'sigmoid'-shaped left ventricle (Dr Jesse Edwards' terminology) or, in my descriptive words, the 'offset' left ventricle-aortic root?

(15) What is the relative importance of the onset of obstruction and the onset of mitral regurgitation in producing pulsus bisferiens, and of the role of the mitral reflex in the Brockenbrough–Braunwald phenomenon?

(16) What has echocardiography contributed?

(17) Should early suspect cases, those with a slight murmur, and teenage children with an abnormal electrocardiogram, have extensive haemodynamic studies, and what is the proper protocol for such studies?

(18) Should suspect cases, e.g. young athletes, restrict their activity?

I expect that these are some of the questions that will be discussed by the members of this study group, and the answers should be much more specific than could be reached six or more years ago.

One of the interesting and, I believe, profitable features of the 1964 symposium was the active discussion. The restricted membership of this study group was also designed to allow a sense of intimacy conducive to argument to develop, which in turn should lead to clarification of the problems and to a crystallization of ideas for possible solutions.

## REFERENCE

WOLSTENHOLME, G. E. W. and O'CONNOR, M. (ed.) (1964) *Ciba Fdn Symp. Cardiomyopathies.* London: Churchill.

# CHANGING CONCEPTS OF HYPERTROPHIC OBSTRUCTIVE CARDIOMYOPATHY IN THE LAST DECADE

## J. F. GOODWIN

Unit of Clinical Cardiology, Department of Medicine,
Royal Postgraduate Medical School, Hammersmith Hospital, London

THE last decade saw the recognition of the disease we now call hypertrophic obstructive cardiomyopathy and the documentation of its clinical, haemodynamic, pathological and functional characteristics. Predictably, the first patients to be described were those with severe obstruction of the outflow tract of the left ventricle, simulating aortic valve stenosis. Although the disease appears to have been described by Schminke in 1907, credit for its recognition in a clinical context goes to Brock in 1957. The pathological characteristics were described by Teare in 1958, who originally called it 'asymmetrical hypertrophy of the heart'. He also drew attention to the familial aspects of the condition, and to the tendency to sudden death.

In 1960 Braunwald and co-workers in the United States analysed the disease, giving it the name 'hypertrophic subaortic stenosis'; in London in the same year we described the same condition under a different name: 'obstructive cardiomyopathy' (Goodwin et al. 1960). Many papers from all parts of the world emphasized left ventricular outflow obstruction and the importance of septal hypertrophy. The generalized nature of the ventricular muscle hypertrophy prompted Jules Cohen to suggest that hypertrophy might be a more important aspect of the disorder. His suggestion has proved to be of far-reaching importance, as I think the discussions at this meeting will show, and he and his colleagues published a further and larger series of patients in 1964 under the title of 'hypertrophic obstructive cardiomyopathy' (Cohen et al. 1964). Increasing knowledge of the condition now emphasizes that hypertrophy is indeed even more important than obstruction (which is not always present) and thus the disorder might be better termed 'hypertrophic

4

cardiomyopathy, obstructive or non-obstructive' (Goodwin 1970).

In North America workers have, perhaps wisely, adhered to their original title, possibly feeling that change would be inappropriate when so much still remains to be learnt about the disease.

The characteristic variability of the outflow tract gradients and the fluctuations in the haemodynamics have made measurements and analysis extremely difficult. The pioneer work of Braunwald and co-workers (1964) in showing the effect of inotropic stimulation and reduction in ventricular volume in abolishing and diminishing outflow tract obstruction greatly improved knowledge of the disease. Five years ago the very existence of an obstructive element was questioned by Criley and co-workers (1965), who showed that gradients in systole could be produced by stimulation of the ventricle under a variety of circumstances and were due to squeezing of the catheter by powerfully contracting muscle in the body of the ventricle. The reverberations of the titanic struggle between Baltimore and Washington crossed the Atlantic, but it soon became obvious that both Criley and Braunwald were correct: the latter demonstrating unequivocal true pressure gradients in hypertrophic subaortic stenosis, and the obvious pitfalls of measuring false gradients being made clear by Criley's important work. Nevertheless, strange anomalies persisted. The rapid initial ventricular ejection, which results in 70 per cent or more of the contents being expelled unimpeded in the first half of systole (Ross et al. 1966), greatly lessens the significance of obstruction late in systole, which occurs after the left ventricle has already contracted down to normal residual volume. The confirmation that the end-systolic ventricular volume was reduced, implying over-emptying of the ventricle (Grant et al. 1968), added weight to Criley's arguments.

Attention has been increasingly paid to what may be termed the 'diastolic component' of the disease. The raised end-diastolic pressure in the left ventricle was noted by Cohen and co-workers (1964), while Stewart, Mason and Braunwald (1968) showed that the rate of filling of the left ventricle was reduced. Subsequent work suggests that this is a more important component of the disease than outflow obstruction. Swan and co-workers (1971) showed that symptoms were more clearly related to diastolic pressure than to outflow gradients, and that a number of patients did not have any outflow obstruction even after provocation. Sudden death appeared to be related more to left ventricular end-diastolic hypertension than to any other factor, although Frank and Braunwald (1968) suggested that patients with a long stable course without deterioration in symptoms did better than those with a short course, a finding which seemed to be borne out by the data of Swan and co-workers. In Frank and Braunwald's (1968) series of 126 patients, the older subjects tended to be more severely symptomatic; those who were initially asymptomatic tended to remain thus, while those who had appreciable symptoms might either become worse or die or improve. Frank and Braunwald also noted that sudden death occurred in both the familial and the apparently sporadic forms of the disease. An interesting feature in most of the patients who died suddenly in our series of 100 patients was the short period between onset of symptoms and death (Swan *et al.* 1971; Goodwin 1970).

Atrial fibrillation is known to occur in around 5 to 10 per cent of patients (Frank and Braunwald 1968; Goodwin 1970; Oakley and Goodwin 1971). We have described a pattern of progression of the disease in some patients which may lead to congestive heart failure. Progressive increase in resistance to ventricular filling leads to increasing left atrial load, reduction in forward output, progressive dyspnoea, and eventually right ventricular failure. The signs of outflow tract obstruction, if present initially, gradually become less and finally disappear. The heart becomes increasingly enlarged, due mainly to atrial dilation. Once atrial fibrillation occurs, embolism is very common (Goodwin 1970; Oakley and Goodwin 1971). Death in congestive heart failure or after systolic embolism is now a recognized form of termination which we had not formerly appreciated.

Mitral regurgitation is more common than usually thought, and indeed probably occurs in all patients with outflow obstruction. The obstruction seems to result from apposition of the hypertrophied septum to the anterior cusp of the mitral valve and hypertrophied anterior papillary muscle, in a 'pinch-cock' type of action. It remains to be seen whether mitral regurgitation is the cause of the obstruction, or merely the result, as is usually believed. New techniques of investigation employing ultrasound will improve knowledge in this area (Pridie and Oakley 1970; Popp and Harrison 1969).

Infective endocarditis, not originally thought to be a hazard in this disease, has been shown to occur by Frank and Braunwald (1968) and Vecht and Oakley (1968). The risk is probably greatest when there is appreciable mitral regurgitation and outflow obstruction. The mitral valve is usually the structure infected.

Pregnancy, originally feared as an added hazard, has proved unsuspectedly benign in our experience (Turner, Oakley and Dijon 1968; Swan *et al.* 1971).

The original concept that there were increased amounts of adrenergic tissue in the outflow tract of the left ventricle, put forward by Pearse (1964), has not been finally confirmed, and this aspect, which we had hoped would have been further advanced, has proved somewhat disappointing.

The last decade has seen the development of treatment by beta-adrenergic blockade in addition to surgery. This treatment was originally introduced on the assumption that β-adrenergic blocking drugs would be likely to produce benefit by preventing arrhythmia, inhibiting sudden death, improving angina, and reducing cardiac work. Exciting new work by Webb-Peploe and co-workers (1971) suggests that the β-adrenergic blocking agent practolol lowers left ventricular diastolic pressure on effort and improves cardiac performance. Further work on the effect of practolol on ventricular compliance is in process and the results will be of great interest.

The indications for, and value of, surgical treatment (Morrow *et al.* 1968) continue to be debated, but most workers are agreed that surgery only produces benefit in patients with outflow tract obstruction.

Thus the last decade has, as would be expected, revealed a much wider spectrum of the disease than originally envisaged and many problems have been uncovered as well as many solved. The cause of the disease and its management still remain the major challenges to our endeavours.

## REFERENCES

BRAUNWALD, E., LAMBREW, C. T., HARRISON, D. C. and MORROW, A. G. (1964) In *Ciba Fdn Symp. Cardiomyopathies*, pp. 172–188. London: Churchill.

BRAUNWALD, E., MORROW, A. G., CORNELL, W. P., AYGEN, M. M. and
    HILLBISH, T. F. (1960) *Am. J. Med.* **29**, 924.

BROCK, R. C. (1957) *Guy's Hosp. Rep.* **106**, 221.

COHEN, J., EFFAT, H., GOODWIN, J. F., OAKLEY, C. M. and STEINER, R. E.
    (1964) *Br. Heart J.* **26**, 16.

CRILEY, J. M., LEWIS, K. B., WHITE, R. I. and ROSS, R. S. (1965) *Circulation*
    **32**, 881.

FRANK, S. and BRAUNWALD, E. (1968) *Circulation* **37**, 759.

GOODWIN, J. F. (1970) *Lancet* **1**, 731.

GOODWIN, J. F., HOLLMAN, A., CLELAND, W. P. and TEARE, R. D. (1960)
    *Br. Heart J.* **22**, 169.

GRANT, C., RAPHAEL, M. J., STEINER, R. E. and GOODWIN, J. F. (1968)
    *Cardiovasc. Res.* **4**, 346.

MORROW, A. G., FOGARTY, T. J., HAMNER, H. III and BRAUNWALD, E.
    (1968) *Circulation* **37**, 581.

OAKLEY, C. M. and GOODWIN, J. F. (1971) To be published.

PEARSE, A. G. E. (1964) In *Ciba Fdn Symp. Cardiomyopathies*, pp. 132–164.
    London: Churchill.

POPP, R. L. and HARRISON, D. C. (1969) *Circulation* **40**, 905.

PRIDIE, R. and OAKLEY, C. M. (1970) *Br. Heart J.* **32**, 203.

ROSS, J. J., BRAUNWALD, E., GAULT, J. H., MASON, D. T. and MORROW,
    A. G. (1966) *Circulation* **34**, 558.

SCHMINKE, A. (1907) *Dt. med. Wschr.* **33**, 2082.

STEWART, S., MASON, D. T. and BRAUNWALD, E. (1968) *Circulation* **37**, 8.

SWAN, D. A., BELL, B. B., OAKLEY, C. M. and GOODWIN, J. F. (1971)
    *Br. Heart J.* in press.

TEARE, R. D. (1958) *Br. Heart J.* **20**, 1.

TURNER, G. M., OAKLEY, C. M. and DIJON, H. G. (1968) *Br. med. J.* **4**, 281.

VECHT, R. J. and OAKLEY, C. M. (1968) *Br. med. J.* **1**, 455.

WEBB-PEPLOE, M., CROXSON, R. S., OAKLEY, C. M. and GOODWIN, J. F.
    (1971) To be published.

# HYPERTROPHIC OBSTRUCTIVE CARDIOMYOPATHY —PATTERNS OF PROGRESSION

## C. M. Oakley

*Unit of Clinical Cardiology, Department of Medicine,
Royal Postgraduate Medical School, Hammersmith Hospital, London*

AFTER more than a decade the student of hypertrophic obstructive cardiomyopathy (HOCM) remains puzzled about many aspects of the disorder but no longer in doubt that it is a progressive disease. At the Royal Postgraduate Medical School, London, we have now studied 105 patients with HOCM. An analysis of the symptomatic course and prognosis of these patients has recently been carried out by Swan and co-workers (1971).

Twenty-four of the 105 patients have died. There have been 14 deaths among the 81 medically treated patients and seven early and three late post-operative deaths among the 24 patients who were treated surgically.

Two deaths were from infective endocarditis (including one of the previously operated patients). Two deaths were associated with cerebral embolism following the onset of atrial fibrillation (including one previously operated patient). Three patients died in congestive heart failure and three other patients who died had developed pulmonary oedema which was the direct cause of death in one. Nine of the 24 deaths were sudden and unexpected (including one of the previously operated patients).

Seventy-three of the 81 surviving patients with HOCM have remained clinically stable but electrocardiographic progression has been notable in a number of these. Not unexpectedly, 'stability' has mainly been a feature of those patients who have been followed for the shortest time.

The changes which developed in 15 of our patients illustrate the possible modes of progression in HOCM. We do not believe that these patients displayed unusual features but rather that they exemplify the usual expectation of patients with HOCM who escape the dangers of infective endocarditis, surgical resection or sudden death at earlier stages of their disease and who are observed

9

over a long period. These, therefore, were patients who did not die 'suddenly' although five of the 15 eventually succumbed to their disease.

We have been recognizing the condition since 1958 and have virtually completed follow-up on the patients but from this experience it is still not possible to make generalizations about the life course of the disease, the rate of progression or the proportion of patients who share the various different clinical syndromes or pass through them. We do not know whether the disease process ever burns itself out and becomes arrested.

In Table I the course and risks of HOCM are depicted as they appear in 1970.

## Sudden death

Sudden death can occur at any stage but in our experience it is least common in patients who have the classical disease as originally described, with a left ventricular outflow tract gradient and mitral regurgitation. We have evidence which suggests that this represents a relatively early phase of the disorder and that sudden death is most likely in patients who have a raised left ventricular end-diastolic pressure and in whom outflow tract obstruction and mitral regurgitation may no longer be a prominent feature (Oakley and Goodwin 1971).

## Infective endocarditis

Infective endocarditis has been seen in four of our patients and in two it proved fatal. Diagnosis is often delayed if the patient is known to have heart muscle disease because such patients are erroneously believed not to be susceptible. All four of these patients had well-marked outflow tract gradients and mitral regurgitation with loud murmurs. Probably infection may be sited either in the outflow tract or in the mitral valve apparatus but we believe that the latter is more likely and this location was proved in one of the fatal cases.

## Progressive loss of murmurs

A spontaneous and progressive decrease in the prominence of the cardiac murmurs was noteworthy in eight patients (Fig. 1). The change was not associated with improvement. Dyspnoea increased, the atrial beat became more forceful

TABLE I

POSSIBLE MECHANISMS OF ONSET AND PROGRESSION IN HYPERTROPHIC OBSTRUCTIVE CARDIOMYOPATHY

### THE PRIMARY FAULT

| *Likely* | *Less favoured* | *Abandoned* |
|---|---|---|
| Congenital predisposition | Truly congenital | Abnormal pathway of ventricular activation |
| 'Hypertrophic muscular dystrophy' (true myopathy) | Primary obstruction | 'Noradrenosis' |
| | Disorder of growth | Super hypertrophy |
| | Metabolic defect | |

### MODE OF PROGRESSION

| *Main features at different phases and their mechanism* | *Clinical presentation* | *Life risks* |
|---|---|---|
| I *Mitral regurgitation and obstruction* — The location of the hypertrophy itself brings about both the obstruction and the regurgitation | 'Classical' (pseudoaortic stenosis etc.) | Infective endocarditis Surgical resection |
| II *Loss of compliance* — Ischaemic fibrosis from increased metabolic demand | Pseudo mitral stenosis | 'Sudden' death Atrial fibrillation Embolism |
| III *Loss of obstruction* — Progression of dystrophic process | Mimicking congestive cardiomyopathy or ischaemic heart disease | Pulmonary oedema |
| IV *Loss of ejectile force* | | Congestive failure |

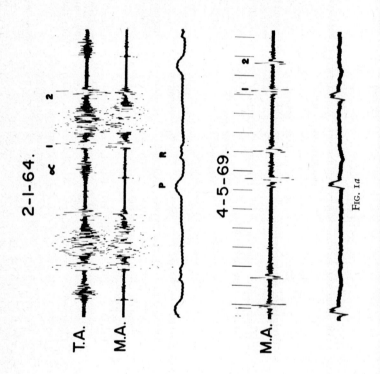

FIG. I*a*

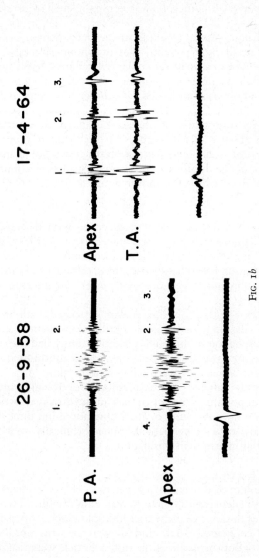

FIG. 1. Spontaneous loss of murmurs in two patients. In both cases the murmurs disappeared before the onset of atrial fibrillation.

FIG. 1b

and progressive cardiomegaly was common but not invariable (Figs. 2 to 4).

These changes were a prelude to the development of atrial fibrillation in all eight patients, four of whom have now died after a period of treatment for congestive failure. Twelve other patients who have never had murmurs or outflow tract obstruction since our observation started have shown no change and one such is illustrated in Fig. 3. This suggests that although loss of the outflow tract obstruction accompanies waning left ventricular powers, its absence *ab initio* carries no such sinister prognosis. The implication is that outflow tract obstruction is not an invariable feature of the disorder at any stage, nor does its continued presence or absence have prognostic significance.

## Dysrhythmias

Progression in ten patients was associated with the onset of atrial fibrillation which was at first intermittent in at least eight of them. One other patient who subsequently died elsewhere with embolism and heart failure had almost certainly had paroxysmal atrial fibrillation but this was never documented with certainty.

The onset of atrial fibrillation was associated with loss of murmurs indicating loss of both outflow obstruction and of mitral regurgitation in those who had previously had these, but the dysrhythmia was also preceded by loss of murmurs in four of the patients while they were still in sinus rhythm.

Six patients suffered systemic embolism, so anticoagulant therapy is important. One patient has survived 12 years without deterioration since the onset of atrial fibrillation, but three other patients have died. Five patients remain clinically well with established or intermittent fibrillation.

## Heart failure

Heart failure was seen in 12 patients. Three patients had pulmonary oedema and all three were in sinus rhythm. Two died as a result of this, one of them after multiple attacks. Six patients went into congestive failure and all were in atrial fibrillation. Dilatation of both atria and of the right ventricle were marked in the patients with congestive heart failure but dilatation of the left ventricle did not usually occur.

*Electrocardiographic changes*

Apart from the development of atrial fibrillation progressive distortion of the electrocardiogram (ECG) occurred over the years. Prolongation of the QRS, the development of fascicular block, the appearance of pathological Q waves and of left and right atrial hypertrophy were seen. Figs. 5 and 6 show the ECG progression in three patients. ECG's which would ordinarily be regarded as diagnostic of infarction were seen in eight patients with HOCM (Fig. 5). The 'infarct' was always anteroseptal in site and was often associated with a left anterior hemiblock type of conduction defect. Septal Q waves were first noted by Wigle who ascribed them to septal fibrosis in 1964. Selective coronary angiography was carried out in nine patients with HOCM including four with pseudo-infarction ECG's, and the coronary arteries were uniformly large in calibre, smooth-walled and free from atheroma. One patient with this ECG pattern was examined at post-mortem. There was no visible focal septal fibrosis but it is true that the septal 'hypertrophe' contains more bulk of muscle, more abnormal muscle and more microscopic interstitial fibrosis than is usually seen in the free wall of the left ventricle. Coyne attributed these ECG changes to a change in spatial orientation of the septum (1968). Both Wigle and Coyne are likely to be right.

*The influence of surgical intervention in the patterns of progression in HOCM*

There are at present 14 survivors of 24 operations for HOCM. All the operations were carried out 'for relief of outflow tract obstruction' in patients with severe symptoms who were thought to have a particularly poor prognosis. The three late postoperative deaths were sudden and unexpected (one patient), from infective endocarditis (one patient) and from heart failure and embolism (one patient). After the apparently striking symptomatic and haemodynamic benefit in two patients and early optimism (Bentall *et al.* 1965), I am now doubtful whether surgical treatment has materially influenced the course of the disease in the others. This belief is the more cogent since loss of obstruction is clearly associated with myocardial deterioration when it occurs naturally and postoperative investigation of the early surgical patients was directed mainly to documentation of outflow tract gradients.

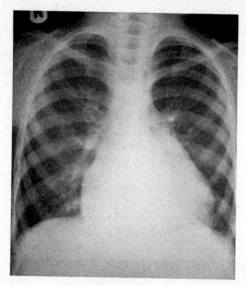

FIG. 2a

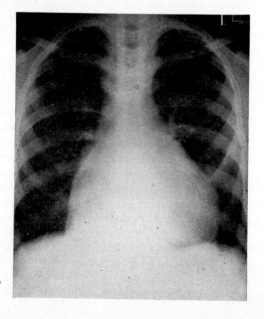

FIG. 2b

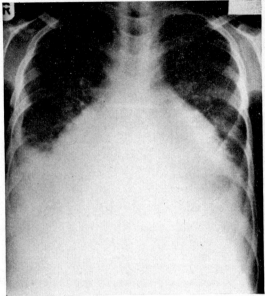

Fig. 2c

Fig. 2. Progressive increase in heart size in the patient (J.H.) whose phonocardiogram is shown in Fig. 1a. The chest radiographs were taken in 1962, 1967 and in 1969 shortly before he died at the age of 18. At autopsy there was a pericardial effusion and slight dilatation of the left ventricular cavity in addition to gross hypertrophy of the septum.

## Mode of onset

We do not yet know the mode of onset of the left ventricular disorder in HOCM. Strong circumstantial evidence suggests that it is usually only the predisposition rather than the disease which is congenital. The minority of patients who present in the first decade usually have the disease in a singularly severe and fatal form. The majority are symptom-free until the third or fourth decade. ECG's and chest radiographs obtained retrospectively have been normal in patients who presented 10 or 20 years later with the fully developed disease.

The reasons for earlier mistaken emphasis on clinical stability

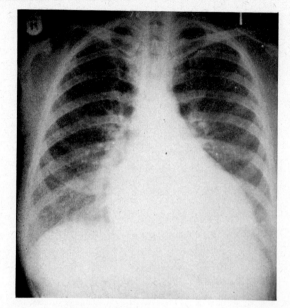

FIG. 3a

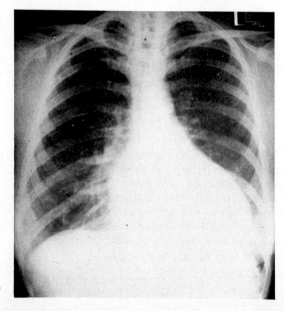

FIG. 3b

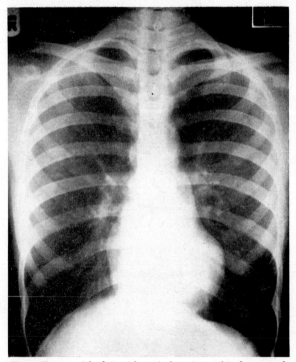

Fig. 4. From a girl of 18 with typical angiographic features of HOCM, no murmurs or outflow tract obstruction and an end-diastolic pressure of 35 mm Hg in the left ventricle.

interrupted by sudden death are easy to understand. These are: (1) the necessarily short period of surveillance possible since the 'birth' of the disease; (2) failure to observe patients during their passage through a time of overt change, e.g. the onset of atrial fibrillation or congestive failure; (3) lack of familiarity with the

Fig. 3. From a woman of 45 who presented with a cerebral embolus and arterial fibrillation in 1958. Her clinical state is still unchanged (chest radiographs 1958 and 1968). The left ventricle is hypertrophied but not dilated; its end-diastolic pressure was 20 mm Hg but there was no outflow tract gradient and she has never had murmurs since we have known her. This patient's 20-year-old daughter had 'classical' HOCM.

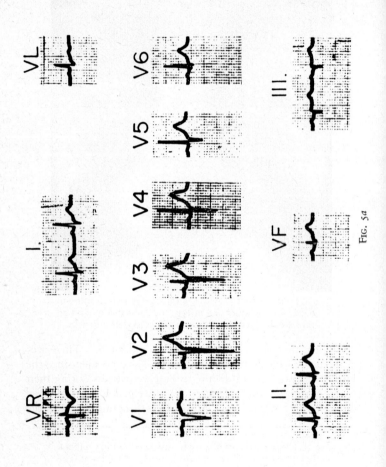

FIG. 5a

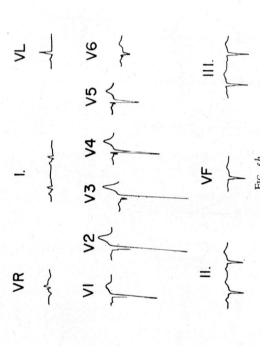

FIG. 5b

FIG. 5. ECG's from a patient who presented with severe left ventricular outflow tract obstruction and pulmonary oedema in 1968. Fig 5b shows left anterior hemiblock and septal Q waves suggest anteroseptal infarction. In 1954 (Fig. 5a) he had a murmur but the ECG and chest radiograph were normal. At autopsy in 1969 the coronary arteries were normal.

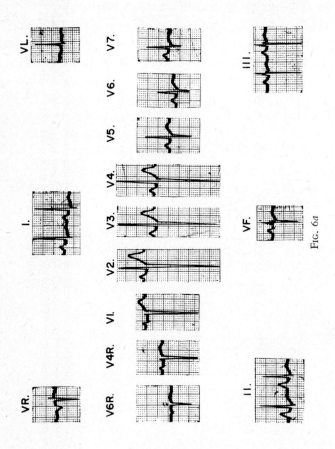

FIG. 6a

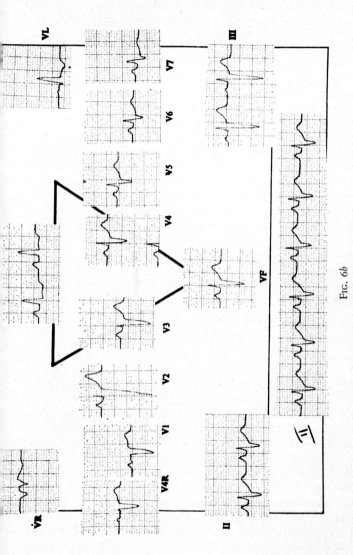

Fig. 6. ECG's at the ages of 11 (a) and 23 years (b) showing typical progression of intraventricular conduction defect in a woman with familial HOCM who has never shown evidence of outflow tract obstruction.

Fig. 6b

diverse clinical guises of the disorder; (4) failure to appreciate that these widely differing clinical and haemodynamic appearances could also be exhibited by individual patients during the lifetime of their disease.

The disorder has been viewed as an abnormality of the anterior mitral papillary muscle which by moving into the left ventricular outflow pathway could determine both obstruction and mitral regurgitation (Oakley *et al.* 1967; Goodwin 1970). It was suggested that the mitral reflux could itself increase obstruction by decompressing the ventricle, thus causing excessive emptying, but this now seems less probable since the leak mainly occurs in late systole after the onset of the obstruction. Mitral echo-cardiography (Fig. 7) carried out for the past two years shows that the anterior cusp reopens in mid-systole after normal systolic closure and at the time of commencement of obstruction it can be seen to approach the septum (Pridie and Oakley 1970; Shah, Gramiak and Kramer 1969; Popp and Harrison 1969). Why the valve should re-open during mid-ejection we do not know but an anatomical cause now seems more likely than an electrophysio-logical one such as could result from mis-routing of the contraction stimulus.

## Left ventricular function

Early recognition of the rapidly rising 'hyperkinetic' arterial pulses (Brachfeld and Gorlin 1959), measurement of a rapid rise of pressure within the left ventricle (high $dp/dt$ max) and the finding of increased left ventricular ejection fractions with a re-duced residual volume of blood all gave an illusion of heightened left ventricular contractile force. The hint of increased myo-cardial resources of noradrenaline (Pearse 1964), now unconfirmed, together with the obvious increase in bulk, gave further support to this misapprehension. When compared with normal hyper-trophied myocardium the increased girth of the myofibrils in HOCM was consistent with 'super' hypertrophy but their disarrangement and malalignment were not. Electron microscopy gave a much clearer picture of sick, deteriorating myofibrils which at first seemed to be at variance with their performance.

Early studies of the disorder were everywhere largely confined to patients with outflow obstruction because this was the criterion by which the disease was recognized. These were patients whose myocardial disease was not yet advanced. The impression of ventricular hyperkinesia in such patients is of course largely spurious since it is the late obstruction to ejection which determines the systolic dip in the arterial pulses and it is fall-off rather than upstroke which is fast. When outflow obstruction is absent the arterial pulses are normal. The rate of rise of pressure in the left ventricle remains normal until late in the disease because the ability of the myofibril to shorten is retained until late in the disease. In fact no patient with HOCM and a dilated left ventricle has yet been studied although one has been seen at post-mortem. Indeed apparent inability to dilate ensures either death or retention of reasonably good ejectile function! Since the ventricle does not dilate, loss of contractile ability obviously results in gross curtailment of output. The loss of cardiac output is particularly severe since increasing slowness of ventricular filling (Stewart, Mason and Braunwald 1968) precedes the contractile failure and negates benefit from a rise in heart rate. The result is an almost inflexible heart rate, stroke volume and minute output, and one such patient with an ejection fraction of $0 \cdot 3$ and end-diastolic volume of $180$ ml/m$^2$ was virtually impervious to all attempts to alter the haemodynamics by the usual pharmacological and physical manoeuvres. Probably the bulky incompliant and fibrotic ventricle is in most instances physically incapable of dilating, so that death is determined rather earlier in the process of contractile power failure than would otherwise be the case. Thus few patients survive to phase IV, but many have now been studied in phases II and III of loss of ventricular distensibility and obstruction (see Table I).

The observation that clinical deterioration is associated with a progressively rising left ventricular filling pressure showed that the major problem in HOCM is loss of myocardial distensibility. The effectiveness of any mode of treatment therefore needs to be judged by its effect on the filling properties of the left ventricle.

Dr Webb-Peploe's studies with practolol have shown the unique response of the left ventricle in HOCM towards beta-sympathetic blockade when compared with the response of the left ventricle in congestive cardiomyopathy or ischaemic heart disease (Webb-Peploe et al. 1971). A *fall* in the raised left ventricular end-diastolic pressure without significant change in end-diastolic volume or ejectile force seems to offer undeniable

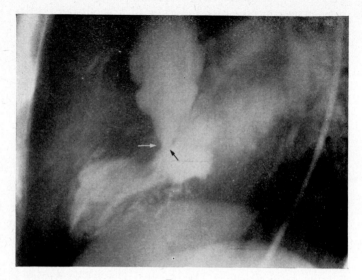

Fig. 7a

Fig. 7. Left ventricular angiogram (a) and mitral echocardiogram (b) in HOCM with outflow tract obstruction and
mitral regurgitation. The echocardiogram shows systolic
reopening (arrowed), the close proximity of the septum at this
time (opposite arrows) and a rather slow diastolic closure rate.
Fig. 7b shows the left ventricle in mid-systole. An abnormal
forward position of the anterior cusp of the mitral valve is
well seen and almost touches the hypertrophied septum
(arrows). This appearance is mirrored on the echocardiogram where the abnormal systolic opening brings the anterior
cusp and septal echoes into apposition. In patients without
outflow tract obstruction or mitral regurgitation (Fig. 7c) the
echocardiogram shows the slow diastolic closure rate
(arrowed) as the sole abnormality. N.B. Downward movements are closing movements of the mitral anterior cusp.
Vertical spots indicate 1 cm excursion. Horizontal spots
indicate time intervals of 0·5 s.

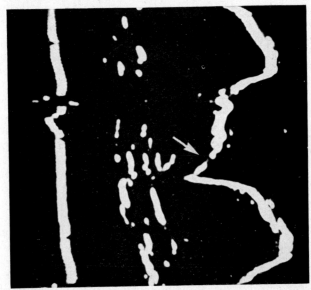

FIG. 7c

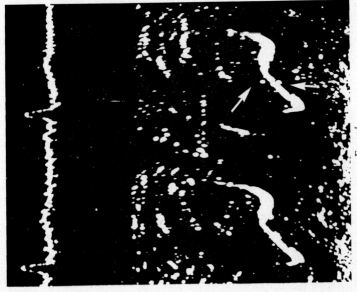

FIG. 7b

evidence of an increase in left ventricular compliance which when combined with maintenance of contractile force and stroke must be therapeutically useful.

These acute studies show that we have a means of controlling the rising left ventricular filling pressure and they gave objective evidence of haemodynamic benefit from β-blockade in HOCM.

Mitral echocardiography at last allows us to follow serial changes in left ventricular performance and the effect of treatment in HOCM, but it is too early yet to say whether long-term oral β-sympathetic blockade really affects the progress and prognosis of the disease.

An abnormal route for ventricular excitation has been postulated to explain left ventricular outflow tract obstruction in HOCM following the theoretical suggestion by the anatomists that premature contraction of the deep bulbospiral muscle could obstruct the outflow tract pathway. Careful plotting of the route of left ventricular depolarization by van Dam, Roos and Durrer (1971) using epicardial electrodes has shown no major fault in HOCM and this again fits in with an acquired rather than a congenital origin of the profound ECG vector abnormalities in HOCM.

In 1969 Meerschwam found abnormal electromyographic potentials from the skeletal muscles of some of his patients with HOCM. These patients had no symptoms or signs of a skeletal myopathy but showed delayed, irregular and polyphasic action potentials and some had raised serum phosphocreatine kinase levels. This had been confirmed in one out of four of our patients who have been similarly studied. Coltart and Meldrum (1970) recently obtained surgical material from the outflow tract of the left ventricle in HOCM and demonstrated striking abnormalities in the action potential of the myofibril. They found grossly delayed repolarization and a reduced velocity of depolarization but a normal resting potential. This exciting new work on the electrophysiology of the myofibril strongly suggests that the myocardial disorder is more akin to a skeletal muscular dystrophy or true myopathy than to a disorder of anatomical growth.

## SUMMARY

Hypertrophic obstructive cardiomyopathy is a progressive disease which causes increasing deterioration in left ventricular performance and the eventual death of the patient. Obstruction to outflow of blood from the left ventricle and mitral regurgitation are features which are commonly but by no means invariably present. Both tend to disappear as myocardial function becomes worse. Both seem to be accidents of the site of hypertrophy and usual location of maximum disease. They are thus incidental to the impaired myocardial performance rather than essential features of the disorder at any stage. Slow ventricular filling at high pressure eventually leads to the development of congestive features often accompanied by atrial fibrillation. Finally, the contractile ability also fails but significant left ventricular dilatation is very rare. Death may occur suddenly at any stage but is commoner in the later phases. Surgery is not beneficial.

Recent work strongly hints that the disorder is a progressive myocardial dystrophy akin to the familial skeletal muscular dystrophies. Hypertrophic myocardial dystrophy is suggested as a suitable name for this disorder.

## REFERENCES

BENTALL, H. H., CLELAND, W. P., OAKLEY, C. M., SHAH, P. M., STEINER, R. E. and GOODWIN, J. F. (1965) *Br. Heart J.* **27**, 585.

BRACHFELD, N. and GORLIN, R. (1959) *Medicine, Baltimore* **38**, 415.

COLTART, D. J. and MELDRUM, S. J. (1970) *Br. med. J.* **4**, 217–218.

COYNE, J. J. (1968) *Br. Heart J.* **30**, 546.

DAM, R. T. VAN, ROOS, J. P. and DURRER, D. (1971) To be published.

GOODWIN, J. F. (1970) *Lancet* **I**, 733.

MEERSCHWAM, I. S. (1969) In *Hypertrophic Obstructive Cardiomyopathy*, p. 129. Amsterdam: Excerpta Medica Foundation.

OAKLEY, C. M. and GOODWIN, J. F. (1971) To be published.

OAKLEY, C. M., RAFTERY, E. B., BROCKINGTON, I. F., STEINER, R. E. and GOODWIN, J. F. (1967) *Br. Heart J.* **29**, 629.

PEARSE, A. G. E. (1964) In *Ciba Fdn Symp. Cardiomyopathies*, pp. 132–164. London: Churchill.

POPP, R. C. and HARRISON, D. C. (1969) *Circulation* **40**, 905.

PRIDIE, R. B. and OAKLEY, C. M. (1970) *Br. Heart J.* **32**, 203.

SHAH, P. M., GRAMIAK, R. and KRAMER, D. H. (1969) *Circulation* **40**, 3–12.

STEWART, S., MASON, D. T. and BRAUNWALD, E. (1968) *Circulation* **37**, 8.

SWAN, D. A., BELL, B. B., OAKLEY, C. M. and GOODWIN, J. F. (1971) *Br. Heart J.* in press.

WEBB-PEPLOE, M., CROXSON, R. S., OAKLEY, C. M. and GOODWIN, J. F. (1971) To be published.

WIGLE, E. D. (1964) In *Ciba Fdn Symp. Cardiomyopathies*, pp. 49–69. London: Churchill.

# THE NATURAL HISTORY OF IDIOPATHIC HYPERTROPHIC SUBAORTIC STENOSIS*

## Eugene Braunwald

*Cardiology Branch, National Heart Institute, Bethesda, Maryland, and Department of Medicine, University of California School of Medicine, San Diego, California*

A total of 126 patients with idiopathic hypertrophic subaortic stenosis (IHSS) have been studied at the National Heart Institute, Bethesda, and most of them have been examined at intervals for up to 12 years. The diagnosis of IHSS was based on a combination of clinical, electrocardiographic, haemodynamic and angio-cardiographic methods as previously outlined (Braunwald *et al.* 1964; Frank and Braunwald 1968). When these 126 patients were first referred to the National Heart Institute, 48 had no limitation of cardiac reserve (Class I), while 50 had symptoms only on exertion (Class II), 25 during mild exertion (Class III), and three at rest (Class IV).

The patients who had more severe symptoms at the initial examination tended to be older (Fig. 1, right), the average age in Class I being 23·7 years, in Class II 31·6 years, and in Classes III and IV 41·1 years. The age at which a heart murmur was first detected (Fig. 1, left), was in many instances the first evidence that heart disease was present. Among the patients who were in Class I when they entered the study, a murmur was first heard at the age of 15·4 years, while in those in Class II it was heard at the age of 20·8 years and at 28·4 years among those in Classes III and IV. Thus, the minimally symptomatic patient with IHSS tended to be younger and to have his murmur detected at an earlier age than the patient with more serious disability.

Also of interest was the similarity in all groups of patients of the time interval between the initial development of symptoms (Fig. 1, centre), or in asymptomatic patients the discovery of a murmur, and the patient's entry into the study. This interval

\* Supported in part by grant HE 12373 from the United States Public Health Service.

averaged 4·4 years in those patients who were least disabled (Class I), 5·2 years in those in Class II, and 6·0 years in those most severely disabled (Classes III and IV). This suggests that

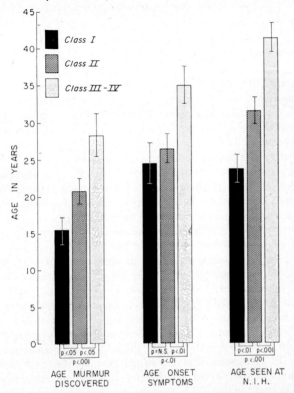

FIG. 1. Age at which a murmur was discovered, age of onset of symptoms, age at which patients were initially seen at N.I.H., and the functional classification at the time of each patient's initial evaluation, according to the New York Heart Association.

mildly and severely symptomatic patients differ more fundamentally than might be anticipated in a single population of patients at different stages of the disease. In the latter case, one would have expected a much longer time interval for the severely disabled as compared to the asymptomatic group. Instead these

2*

findings suggest that two different populations may exist: a younger group of patients who are asymptomatic or mildly disabled, and an older group in whom the clinical manifestations develop later in life and who become progressively more disabled.

*Follow-up studies*

Ninety-eight of the 126 patients in this series have been followed up, some for as long as 12 years (Fig. 2). Forty-two of the 48 patients who were in functional Class I at the time of the initial examination have had one or more re-examinations, with an average follow-up period of 38·2 months, and a total follow-up period of 133·6 patient years. Thirty of these 42 patients (71%) have shown no change in their functional status. One patient, an asymptomatic boy, died suddenly. Eight patients deteriorated clinically, two having recurrent bouts of arrhythmia, while the other six developed angina pectoris, syncope, or symptoms of congestive heart failure. Three of these eight patients were operated upon when their condition worsened. A fluctuating course was noted in the remaining three of the 42.

Forty of the 50 patients who on initial examination were in functional Class II have had one or more re-examinations, with an average follow-up period of 33 months, and a total follow-up period of 110·2 patient-years. The clinical course tended to be much more variable than in those initially in Class I, and only 19 of the 40 (47%) initially in Class II have remained stable and in this class. Five of the 40 patients died between 6 and 53 months after their initial evaluation, three of them unexpectedly; these three patients were in Class II until they died. A fourth patient became Class III 29 months after the initial examination, and died in pulmonary oedema two months later. Another patient gradually deteriorated to Class IV 21 months after her initial examination, and suffered from refractory angina pectoris when she died 30 months later. Five other patients deteriorated during follow-up and they progressed to Class III six to 36 months after entering the study. The remaining 11 patients in Class II exhibited an extremely variable course and their condition has fluctuated considerably during observation. However, none of the patients who were in Class II at the time of entry into the study are now in functional Class I.

Twenty-eight patients were in Classes III or IV at the time of

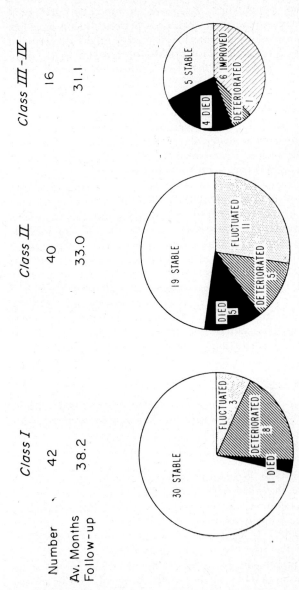

|  | Class I | Class II | Class III - IV |
|---|---|---|---|
| Number | 42 | 40 | 16 |
| Av. Months Follow-up | 38.2 | 33.0 | 31.1 |

FIG. 2. The clinical course of patients in various functional classifications at the time of entry into the study. The patients in Class I tended to remain stable, whereas those who were more disabled (Classes II to IV) tended to pursue a more variable course.

their initial examinations. Seven were promptly operated upon, and five have not yet been followed. Sixteen patients have had one or more re-examinations for an average follow-up period of 31 months, representing a total follow-up period of 41·5 patient years. Four of these 16 died, two of them in refractory heart failure and two suddenly. The condition of five patients has remained stable; four of these were operated upon. One patient deteriorated clinically, progressed from Class III to Class IV, and was then operated upon. Six patients exhibited distinct clinical improvement while under observation. Four of them, initially in Class III, are now in functional Class II, while two are in Class I, 90 and 140 months after entry into the study.

Thus, these observations emphasize the extreme variability of the course of patients with IHSS. In some patients no symptomatic change has occurred for as long as six years; some patients have deteriorated progressively; others showed considerable spontaneous improvement; several patients died of their disease and the remainder pursued a fluctuating course. Despite this variability, the course of those who were asymptomatic or mildly disabled on initial examination was generally stable and they seldom deteriorated during the several years of observation. On the other hand, a significant proportion of the patients who were more seriously disabled at the time of entry into the study died or deteriorated further, and a smaller number improved spontaneously.

### Bacterial endocarditis

In this series of 126 patients, three had documented endocarditis, one had probable and another two had possible bacterial endocarditis.

### Deaths

Fourteen of the 98 patients who have been followed (14%) have died during the course of the study. Four of the 14 deaths cannot be considered to be a direct result of the natural history of IHSS, leaving ten patients who died as a direct consequence of their disease (Table I). In six of these ten patients the deaths were sudden, while the other four became increasingly disabled.

Five of the ten patients whose deaths could be attributed to the natural history of IHSS had the familial form of the disease and the

## Table I
### Deaths by IHSS

| | Pt. no. | Age (years) | | | | Sex | Fam. hx. | LV-art. gradient (mm Hg) | | NYHA class | | Duration of symptoms | | | | | Post-mortem |
|---|---|---|---|---|---|---|---|---|---|---|---|---|---|---|---|---|---|
| | | M | Sx | NIH | Died | | | Basal | $\bar{c}$ Prov. | Init. | Final | Ang. | Syn. | CHF | Palp. | DOE | |
| Sudden deaths | 64 | 4 | — | 7 | 11 | M | Pos | — | I=34 | I | I | — | — | — | — | — | Diagnosis confirmed |
| | 75 | 8 | 8 | 10 | 15 | M | Pos | 30 | — | II | II | 6Y | 5Y | — | — | 7Y | Not performed |
| | 77 | 5 | 7 | 7 | 8 | M | Pos | 15 | — | II | II | — | — | — | — | 9M | Diagnosis confirmed |
| | 43 | 24 | 35 | 40 | 43 | M | Neg | 0 | I=70 V=70 | III | III | 3Y | 3Y | — | — | 8Y | Diagnosis confirmed |
| | 85 | 48 | 48 | 52 | 53 | F | Neg | 0 | I=70 | II | II | — | — | — | 4Y | 4Y | Diagnosis confirmed |
| | 124 | 20 | 25 | 27 | 29 | M | Neg | 74 | — | III | III | 3Y | — | 3Y | — | 3Y | Not performed |
| Progressive deterioration | 8 | 12 | 15 | 28 | 33 | F | Pos | 0 | I=9 V=0 | II | IV | 4Y | 5Y | 4Y | — | 18Y | Diagnosis confirmed |
| | 45 | 26 | 26 | 39 | 41 | F | Neg | 87 | — | III | IV | 4Y | — | 13Y | — | 4Y | Not performed |
| | 53 | 12 | 18 | 25 | 27 | F | Pos | 8 | — | III | IV | — | — | — | 4Y | 9Y | Diagnosis confirmed |
| | 115 | 24 | 32 | 34 | 36 | F | Neg | 75 | V=125 | II | IV | 3Y | — | 2M | 2M | 4Y | Diagnosis confirmed |

Age: M = Age murmur discovered; Sx = Age of onset of symptoms; NIH = age of first admission to NIH. Fam. hx. = family history.

LV-art. gradient = left ventricular-arterial gradient; $\bar{c}$ Prov. = left ventricular-arterial gradient during provocative tests; I = isoproterenol (isoprenaline) infusion; V = Valsalva manoeuvre; (—) = test not performed.

Symptoms: Ang. = angina pectoris; Syn. = syncope; CHF = congestive heart failure; Palp. = palpitations; DOE = dyspnoea on exertion; Y = years; M = months.

other five the sporadic form. Five deaths occurred in males and five in females. The ages at death ranged from eight to 53 years, with an average of 29·6 years. There was no significant difference in the ages of the six patients who died suddenly and the four who died after progressive deterioration, or between the males and the females. However, the five patients with familial IHSS who succumbed did so at a significantly younger age (18·8 years) than the five with the sporadic form of the disease (40·4 years, $P<0·01$).

Only three of the ten patients had serious obstruction to left ventricular outflow (Fig. 3), with peak systolic pressure gradients exceeding 70 mm Hg in the basal state, while the other seven

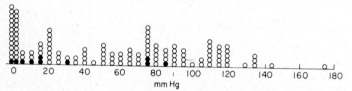

FIG. 3. Peak basal left ventriculo-arterial systolic pressure gradient at the time of the initial catheterization. Only three of the 10 patients who died of IHSS had a systolic pressure gradient exceeding 30 mm Hg.

patients had either no detectable or only mild obstruction, with peak systolic pressure gradients in the basal state ranging from zero to 30 mm Hg; two of the latter developed severe obstruction with provocation. At the time of death only one of the ten patients, an 11-year-old boy with familial IHSS, was totally asymptomatic; three patients were in functional Class II, two in Class III, and four in Class IV. Six of the ten had suffered from angina pectoris, and three had experienced syncopal episodes and palpitations. Nine had complained of dyspnoea on exertion and five had been in congestive heart failure. The fear that sudden death may occur and the impression that it may be due to severe obstruction to left ventricular outflow has in the past led to operative treatment being recommended for an increasing number of asymptomatic or only mildly disabled patients with no or slight obstruction, particularly those with the familial form of IHSS. The findings of the present study do not support such a course of action.

*Pressure measurements*

In the basal state the peak systolic pressure gradient between the left ventricle and either the aorta or brachial artery ranged from zero to 175 mm Hg, with an average value of 54·3 mm Hg (Fig. 3). The patients with familial IHSS had gradients which were significantly lower (average 42·4 mm Hg) than the patients with the sporadic form of the disease (average 60·4 mm Hg; $P < 0.05$) (Fig. 4, left). The average gradients in the patients in functional Class I (48·0 mm Hg) and Class II (51·8 ± 5·6 mm Hg) were not significantly different. However, the average gradient in the patients in Classes III and IV (70·7 mm Hg) was significantly higher ($P < 0.05$) than in those in Class I (Fig. 4, centre). All four patients in whom the pressure gradient increased significantly on serial left heart catheterization also deteriorated clinically.

The left ventricular end-diastolic pressure was abnormally high ($> 12$ mm Hg) in approximately three-fourths of the patients, but this did not correlate with either the degree of disability or with the familial or sporadic nature of the disease. Significant obstruction to right ventricular outflow, defined as a peak systolic pressure gradient exceeding 10 mm Hg in the basal state, was observed in only 15 per cent of the patients.

*Cardiac output*

The cardiac index for the entire group of patients averaged 3·15 l/min per square metre of body surface area. Eleven patients (9%) had indices lower than 2·00 l/min m$^{-2}$, and 16 (14%) had indices exceeding 4·00 l/min per square metre. The average cardiac index in the 42 patients in Class I (3·65 l/min m$^{-2}$) was significantly higher than in the 49 in Class II (2·88 l/min m$^{-2}$; $P < 0.01$) or in the 27 in classes III and IV (2·79 l/min m$^{-2}$; $P < 0.01$) (Fig. 4, right). There was no significant difference between the average cardiac index in the patients with the familial and the sporadic forms of the disease.

*Familial versus sporadic forms of IHSS*

Forty of the 126 patients (32%) were considered to have familial IHSS, while 86 (68%) had the sporadic form of the disease. Patients with familial IHSS were younger (average 26·8 years) than those with the sporadic form of the disease (average 32·7 years; $P < 0.05$) (Fig. 5), and there was a higher

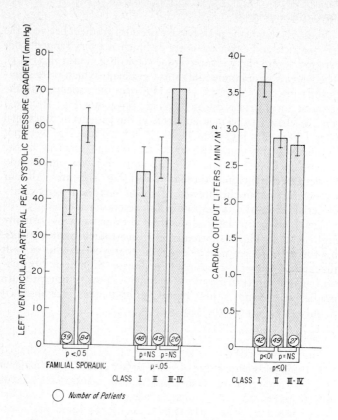

Fig. 4. Haemodynamic observations in IHSS. Left: the ventriculo–arterial peak systolic pressure gradients in patients with familial IHSS and those with the sporadic form of the disease. The columns represent the mean value ± 1 standard error. Centre: a comparison of peak systolic pressure gradients in patients in functional Classes I, II, and III–IV. P=NS, indicates no significant difference. Right: a comparison of the cardiac output in patients in Classes I, II, and III–IV.

incidence of females in the familial (18 of 40, 45%) than in the sporadic form (24 of 86, 28%). The sporadic form of IHSS was uncommon in girls and young women, while familial IHSS was rare in older men. Females with IHSS tended to be more severely disabled.

Neither the physical findings nor the clinical course (Fig. 6) could be correlated with the familial or sporadic nature of the

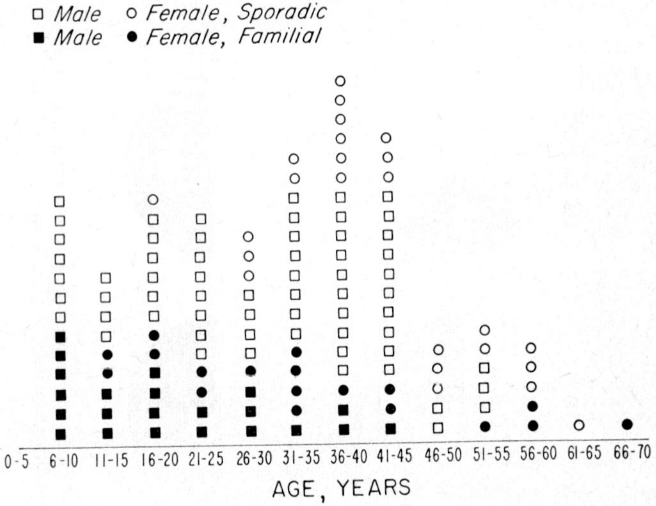

FIG. 5. The age, sex, and family incidence in IHSS. Each symbol denotes one patient. Note the relatively small number of young females with sporadic IHSS and of older males with familial IHSS.

disease. The mortality rates did not differ significantly. In each group three patients died unexpectedly, and two succumbed after chronic cardiac decompensation. Patients with the familial form of IHSS had a higher incidence of right axis deviation or indeterminate axis (6 of 39, 15%) in contrast to the extremely unusual occurrence of this finding in the sporadic form (2 of 84, 2%; $P < 0.01$). The incidence of intraventricular conduction defects was significantly higher in familial patients (13 of 39, 33%) than in those with the sporadic form (9 of 84, 11%; $P < 0.005$), and electrocardiographic evidence of left ventricular hypertrophy was seen less often in the patients with familial IHSS (21 of 39 patients, 54%) than in those with the sporadic form (65 of 84, 77%; $P < 0.02$). The difference in the severity of obstruction in the two groups has already been commented upon.

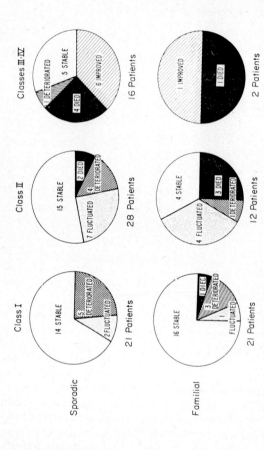

FIG. 6. The clinical course of IHSS according to the functional class of the patient at the time of entry into the study and the familial or sporadic nature of the disease.

## SUMMARY

While much information about the haemodynamic and angiographic features of idiopathic hypertrophic subaortic stenosis (IHSS) is available, data on the natural history of the disease are limited. The clinical courses of 126 patients with haemodynamically documented IHSS, examined repeatedly for up to 12 years, were analysed. The older patients tended to be more severely symptomatic. Although the course was extremely variable, the patients who were asymptomatic initially tended to remain so, while those who were more disabled generally deteriorated, died, or improved spontaneously. Ten patients died as a consequence of the natural history of IHSS; six of these deaths were unexpected. Sudden deaths occurred usually in patients with no or mild obstruction, and in patients with both the familial and sporadic forms of the disease.

## REFERENCES

BRAUNWALD, E., LAMBREW, C. T., ROCKOFF, S. D., ROSS, J. JR and MORROW, A. G. (1964) *Circulation* **29**, Suppl. IV, IV–1.
FRANK, S. and BRAUNWALD, E. (1968) *Circulation* **37**, 759–788.

## DISCUSSION

*Burchell:* Both Professor Goodwin and Dr Oakley significantly have referred to '*the* disease' of hypertrophic obstructive cardiomyopathy (HOCM) in the singular, thus indicating their belief in a unitary cause of the problem.

*Meerschwam:* When the family history of a patient with HOCM includes relatives who showed heart disability or who died suddenly at an early age, there is no difficulty in classifying the case as a familial one. But where there is no such history, one still cannot say this is a sporadic case, especially in a disease which often may be asymptomatic. In our first series of 23, three patients whom we thought were sporadic cases with completely sound family histories, after thorough family investigation turned out to have close relatives showing distinct clinical, electrocardiographic and phonocardiographic signs pointing to the presence of the disease. Classification of sporadic and familial cases only on the basis of the history may therefore be dangerous.

*Braunwald:* It could certainly be dangerous but in every instance we examined all available close relatives of our patients very carefully, bringing some from as far as 3000 miles away for study. We often carried out haemodynamic studies in these relatives to determine the presence or absence of the disease. But having said that, I agree with you that one can only be certain of the familial or non-familial nature of the disease in the former group. So, if anything, the differences between these two groups are greater than we indicated because the non-familial group was probably 'contaminated' with patients with familial disease, even though we went to great lengths to track down the relatives.

*Nellen:* Out of about 150 patients in South Africa we have seen only one definite case in an African, and one other possible one. Is there any such difference between the negro and the white population in America?

*Braunwald:* Although there were several negroes in our series, the number was far less than 10 per cent, which corresponds to the fraction of negroes in the total U.S. population.

*Nellen:* Did the 20 per cent or so of your patients who had no obstruction even at rest or on provocation have systolic murmurs?

*Braunwald:* No. These patients presented simply with left ventricular hypertrophy and if they had not had a family history of myocardial hypertrophy with the accident of obstruction they would have been classified as having idiopathic myocardial hypertrophy and not as having IHSS.

*Shah:* I find it difficult to agree with the view proposed by Dr Oakley and associates that outflow obstruction is an incidental finding in the disease and of little consequence in the clinical determination of a patient. Among the evidence contradicting such a hypothesis are Dr Braunwald's studies correlating the outflow gradients with the clinical state, and postoperative follow-up studies from several centres that clearly correlate the clinical improvement with relief of outflow gradients. Since it is well known that the presence and the degree of outflow obstruction can be quite variable in a given patient, depending largely on the inotropic state and intraventricular volumes, I would like to ask Dr Oakley whether haemodynamic studies were undertaken in patients with clinical deterioration in whom the murmur was absent. Could the obstruction be provoked by the usual physiological and pharmacological manoeuvres?

*Oakley:* Eight patients lost obstruction but deteriorated in association with rising end-diastolic pressures. I didn't make graphs because the end-diastolic pressures are as variable as the outflow tract gradients. In the same individual on the same study occasion the end-diastolic pressure (LVEDP) can vary between 10 mm Hg at rest and 45 mm Hg on mild exercise! This makes it exceedingly difficult to make valid comparisons between the results of haemodynamic studies carried out on different occasions. Clinically it is much easier: the development of unequivocal radiological signs of pulmonary venous congestion when these were previously absent is fairly acceptable evidence. Haemoptysis occurred in two of the patients. Atrial fibrillation and systemic congestion followed in three of them. The fallacy inherent in displaying 'spot' measurements for LVEDP is illustrated by one of our early patients whose 'spot' (post-A wave) LVEDP was 45 mm Hg when he was first studied. He then had no severe dyspnoea or radiological abnormality in the lung fields to suggest a persistently elevated pulmonary venous pressure. Six years later when there was floridly obvious pulmonary congestion with haemoptysis and failure the LVEDP was only 15, but he was fibrillating and the stroke volume had greatly diminished. These people are operating on the steep part of their ventricular compliance curves and one really needs accurate volume/pressure measurements throughout diastolic filling before statements about compliance changes can be made.

The haemodynamic correlate is that at the stage of loss of outflow obstruction the left ventricle is beginning to lose its previously well-maintained contractile ability, so the end-systolic volume gets a bit bigger and obstruction ceases to happen through the accident of the bulky septal muscle hitting the anterior cusp during ejection.

*Shah:* I don't believe that my question has been fully answered. Were you able to provoke obstruction in these patients?

*Oakley:* Yes, for a while, but even this may disappear. Again we haven't been able to justify repeating left heart catheterizations in the same individuals on enough occasions to document this haemodynamically. The clinical correlate of this was however very striking. Two patients did show a loud murmur after post-ectopic pauses but then eventually lost this sign, the assumption being that even with the help of post-extrasystolic potentiation the left ventricle failed to empty sufficiently for the 'accident' of outflow tract obstruction to happen any more.

*Burchell:* Does your coding or indexing system include the category of 'idiopathic hypertrophy' or do you group all cases of hypertrophy without valvular disease, hypertension and inflammatory disease as 'cardiomyopathy', classifying them as either inflow or outflow obstruction?

*Oakley:* Our ultimate diagnostic criterion is the end-diastolic volume. Failure of contractile function and ejectile ability with dilatation puts a patient into the congestive cardiomyopathy group, not the HOCM group, unless such a patient has previously been in the HOCM group with an outflow tract gradient and a small left ventricular cavity. We have not yet seen this happen, although if a patient with HOCM could dilate up his cavity he would survive longer. Usually I think they die in the rather early stages of loss of contractile ability because if the diastolic cavity size fails to increase a great fall in stroke volume follows. We no longer recognize a group of idiopathic hypertrophy. The reasons are simple. We have seen patients who have had 'typical HOCM' develop into a phase when they have 'idiopathic hypertrophy'. We have also seen that the relatives of patients with 'typical HOCM' may have 'idiopathic hypertrophy', as Dr Braunwald has already mentioned. This seems to be a functional distinction without an aetiological difference. I am an unrepentant 'lumper'.

If we make an analogy with the skeletal myopathies, there are different modes of inheritance, different somatic locations of the myopathy and different rates of progression. The only trend of difference we could find between familial and sporadic cases was that patients with a family history sometimes presented earlier and fared worse. There was no detectable point of difference between the patients who presented with 'idiopathic hypertrophy' and those who progressed into this category after having gone through a phase of outflow tract obstruction.

*Wigle:* We have analysed the clinical course of 60 patients with hypertrophic cardiomyopathy, all of whom had outflow tract obstruction. In 20 per cent the family history was positive. Of the 60 patients, 27 initially had no treatment and ten have remained untreated; 13 were initially treated and 21 finally treated with propranolol; 20 initially and 32 eventually underwent surgery.

We carried out both retrospective and prospective studies on our patients. Of the ten untreated patients, three have died, two of them from the disease, and one patient has been lost to follow-up. Apart from this patient, of the 27 initially untreated patients 26 remained untreated for a total follow-up of 104 patient-years, with an average follow-up of four years. Of the eight patients who were Class I (asymptomatic) on the New York Heart Association classification two remained thus, one deteriorated to Class II, four to Classes III–IV, and one died. Of the nine patients who began in Class II four remained the same, four deteriorated to III–IV and one died. Of those in Class III some deteriorated to IV and one died. Thus we have a picture of a gradually progessive deterioration in these patients with hypertrophic cardiomyopathy and outflow tract obstruction. The murmur was first noted at a mean age of 21 years (range 0–46 years), with the onset of mild symptoms (Class II, N.Y.H.A.) by age 31 (range 2–50) and severe symptoms (Class III) at age 36 (range 12–56). If we add the 11 haemodynamically proved cases of muscular subaortic stenosis from the Hospital for Sick Children in Toronto (because the Toronto General is an adult hospital), the average age at which murmur was noted goes down to 17 and the age of onset of symptoms was slightly lower (18 years). In the familial cases the murmur was noted at an average age of 19 years and the average age of onset of symptomatology was 26 years.

The natural history of our cases with obstruction to outflow was that mild symptoms commenced an average of ten years after the murmur was noted, and more severe symptoms (Class III) five years later. Five of 28 non-surgically treated patients died an average of five years after the onset of Class III symptomatology. Of course, sudden death can occur at any time. In analysing the haemodynamic parameters of the patients in the different functional classes of the N.Y.H.A. classification, there was a progressive rise in left ventricular end-diastolic pressure and a fall in cardiac index as the symptomatology became more severe, but these differences were not statistically significant. The patients with Class III–IV symptomatology however had a significantly greater degree of outflow tract obstruction than patients in Class II ($P < 0.05$).

*Burchell:* Dr Olsen, do pathologists still distinguish hearts as having septal hypertrophy or diffuse hypertrophy, in the two categories of familial or sporadic?

*Olsen:* I will be discussing that later (see pp. 183–191).

Dr Braunwald, did you find any pathological differences between the sporadic and the familial type?

*Braunwald:* No, we did not.

*Olsen:* Both Professor Goodwin and Dr Oakley hinted that this might be a myocardial disease. In the present state of our knowledge and with the methods of investigation so far used, we have come to the conclusion that there are definite abnormal cells which can be recognized. I think the various clinical manifestations can be explained partly by the distribution of the aggregates of these abnormal myocardial fibres. The bulk of the myocardium, however, shows hypertrophy which is in no way different from the secondary change whenever left ventricular hypertrophy takes place.

*Emanuel:* Dr Braunwald, would you elaborate the evidence for suggesting there may be a different aetiology in the familial and sporadic forms of this disease?

*Braunwald:* By definition in the familial cases we are clearly dealing with a familial disease and in the truly non-familial cases we are not. With the exceptions I have noted, however, both groups had similar clinical manifestations.

*O'Brien:* Were any of the deaths in your patients known to be associated with arrhythmias of either short onset or prolonged duration? While I was at the National Institutes of Health we had 15 patients who had atrial fibrillation and, possibly in contrast to Dr Oakley's patients, in most it was a very dramatic deterioration (Glancy *et al.* 1970). Secondly all these 15 patients had obstruction which persisted even though they had atrial fibrillation. Furthermore, in atrial fibrillation when there is a long diastolic pause the subsequent beat is associated with an increased gradient, so at least in this circumstance increased volume is not associated with decreased obstruction.

*Braunwald:* In two of the ten who died as a direct consequence of their disease death was associated with arrhythmia, in one patient for a short period and in one for a longer period before death. At the time of your analysis, Dr O'Brien, the number of patients had grown and the number that fell into this category had grown as well.

*Burchell:* There is also the question of potentiation following a short cycle.

*Brock:* I was particularly impressed with your comment, Professor Burchell, that everybody is talking about '*a*' disease or '*the* disease' although it is by no means clear that it is one disease. Apart from that, an aspect I would like to introduce is that the recognition of the condition first of all came from the clinical importance and recognition of outflow tract obstruction. Dr Wigle emphasized the dominance of that and Dr Oakley has now introduced the later recognition of the importance of inflow obstruction. As I see it, we are all certainly talking about a condition which is called idiopathic cardiomyopathy, or obstructive cardiomyopathy, and we have squeezed out a tremendous amount of clinical, pathological and other information about it. But other aspects of the function of the left ventricle have got to be considered, both from the point of view of differential diagnosis and because they may shed light upon the condition itself.

I am interested therefore in those conditions which occur as a result of obstruction of the left ventricular outflow tract, particularly those in which there is an organic obstruction. We agree that there is a variable distribution of the hypertrophic changes and therefore in the functional obstruction which may appear in this disease which many of us have selected to discuss exclusively here, but let us consider the patient who has an organic obstruction of the left ventricle. Attention was first directed to this condition because it occurs in the right ventricle as a subvalvular hypertrophy causing obstruction. It seemed by analogy that such a condition could and should occur in the left ventricle, even allowing for physiological and anatomical variations between the two ventricles. I am concerned with the condition occurring with valvular or subvalvular organic obstruction. First of all with valvular aortic stenosis one has to consider the importance of the part played by secondary subvalvular or subaortic obstruction due to hypertrophy of the muscle. In other words this is a localized obstructive condition, not necessarily associated with any diffuse disease of the muscle, although some cases do have a muscular abnormality. This subaortic obstruction can play an important part in the possibility of a fatal complication after valvotomy or valve replacement if one does not recognize that such a functional obstruction may occur. For instance in right ventricular obstruction we often notice that the obstruction is aggravated in the early postoperative phase. I am particularly interested in those cases in which the primary obstruction is an organic subaortic obstruction, a fibrous or fibromuscular hypertrophy. In my naïveté as a surgeon, I have thought that if we cut out a severe organic fibrous obstruction the condition would be cured, but in fact the results can be very disappointing. The organic obstruction can recur or a hypertrophic type of muscular obstruction can occur. A few years ago I did a very satisfactory operation on a child with such a fibrous subvalvular stenosis, and later heard that the Mayo Clinic had done a second satisfactory operation. Now the same patient is going to have another satisfactory operation in Houston. In these children the onset of a hypertrophic type of obstruction secondary to the primary or organic obstruction is a reality and I don't think we have even considered it here. I hope that we shall not overlook this in our general presentation of the matter.

Hywel Davis has written an interesting paper (1970) about four cases of what he calls hypertrophic subaortic stenosis, which we are taught is a bad term now, as a complication of fixed obstruction of left ventricular outflow. He gives examples of near-fatal functional obstruction occurring after operations for both valvular and subaortic stenosis. This paper summarizes very simply the association of these problems with an organic obstruction.

*Goodwin:* I agree entirely with what you say, Lord Brock. There are patients who have muscle hypertrophy indistinguishable from the hypertrophic cardiomyopathies we have been discussing, secondary to a fixed organic outflow obstruction of valve stenosis or discrete subvalvular stenosis. I am equally sure that it is important as regards the condition we have been discussing.

I certainly think we are dealing with one disease and that we do not have the evidence to say there are both sporadic and familial forms. It seems to me that the pathology, the clinical picture and the haemodynamic features all point to there being one condition in which many of the familial cases are hidden. As Dr Oakley says, they haven't yet emerged; they haven't yet developed enough signs of the disease to permit diagnosis. Many of our patients give a family history which strongly suggests that some relative had the disease but we cannot prove it because the evidence is not available.

## REFERENCES

DAVIS, H. (1970) *Guy's Hosp. Rep.* **119,** 35.
GLANCY, D. L., O'BRIEN, K. P., GOLD, H. K. and EPSTEIN, S. E. (1970) *Br. Heart J.* **32,** 652-659.

# THE FAMILIAL INCIDENCE OF IDIOPATHIC CARDIOMYOPATHY

## R. EMANUEL

*National Heart Hospital and Department of Cardiology,
Middlesex Hospital, London*

IN 1947 William Evans in a communication to the British Cardiac Society drew attention to a new clinical entity which featured cardiomegaly, dysrhythmias, including Adam-Stokes attacks, and sudden death. He also noted a familial incidence and proposed the name 'familial cardiomegaly' (Evans 1949). Today these cases would be diagnosed as cardiomyopathy. Since William Evans' original description 23 years ago very little progress has been made in our understanding of the genetics of this disease.

The present state of our knowledge can be summarized by saying that a percentage of the cardiomyopathies, particularly the hypertrophic group, have a familial tendency and when this occurs the defect is transmitted as a non-sex-linked autosomal dominant and the chromosomes are normal.

### MATERIAL AND METHODS

The present study, which was started in October 1967, was undertaken to determine the familial incidence of idiopathic cardiomyopathy. The work, although entering its final stage, is not yet complete.

The propositi, all of whom had proven cardiomyopathies, were patients who had attended the National Heart Hospital, Hammersmith Hospital, or the Middlesex Hospital between 1963 and 1967 inclusive. Clinical assistance and existing data were made available by various colleagues who collaborated in this work. These included J. F. Goodwin, K. A. Hallidie-Smith, A. Kristinsson, E. L. McDonald, C. M. Oakley, J. Somerville and W. Somerville.

Propositi were only accepted when the clinical diagnosis of cardiomyopathy had been confirmed by cardiac catheterization and left ventricular angiography, or by operation or necropsy. A number of cases also had coronary arteriography. Each physician responsible for a propositus was asked to indicate whether the case was 'hypertrophic' or 'congestive', according to the criteria suggested by Goodwin (Goodwin et al. 1961; Goodwin 1964, 1970). Cases in which the aetiology was known were excluded, i.e. cardiomyopathy associated with a collagen disease, amyloid, alcohol, or those cases which were thought to follow a viral myocarditis.

A total of 121 cases of idiopathic cardiomyopathy were seen at the three hospitals. The families of 99 were interviewed and included in the study. The remaining 22 were excluded on the following grounds: nine of the index cases had left the country or could not be traced, seven were unwilling to cooperate, and in five instances, although the propositus was in the United Kingdom the relatives lived abroad, and one of the propositi was adopted. Of the 99 propositi accepted for this study 78 were diagnosed as hypertrophic and 21 as congestive. The families under review consisted of 198 parents, 307 siblings, and 133 children, making a total of 638 first-degree relatives.

The object of the study was to examine all living first-degree relatives and to obtain maximum information about those who had died.

The general practitioner of the propositus was contacted and then an explanatory letter requesting an interview was sent to each family, generally to the propositus. The family was seen at home whenever possible, as it is common experience in this type of work that more accurate family details are collected in the relaxed atmosphere of the home than in hospital surroundings. At the interview a family pedigree was constructed which included all first- and second-degree relatives and first cousins.

All first-degree relatives who were willing to cooperate were examined clinically and had an electrocardiogram and chest radiograph. Whenever possible, examination was arranged at the hospital which the propositus had attended; failing this the local consultant or cardiologist was asked to carry out the examination and his report, together with the electrocardiogram and chest radiograph, was sent to me at the National Heart Hospital.

The diagnosis of cardiomyopathy was only accepted when the physical findings, chest radiograph, and electrocardiogram were all compatible, or when there was operative or necropsy evidence. In a number of relatives, particularly children, it was not possible to be certain of the diagnosis of cardiomyopathy without cardiac catheterization and left ventricular angiography, and this was rarely considered justifiable. These have been grouped separately as 'doubtful' cases. By adopting this conservative attitude we have no doubt underestimated the familial incidence.

RESULTS

The present state of the study is shown in Table I. We anticipate that finally we shall have examined over 85 per cent of all first-degree relatives.

TABLE I

PRESENT STATE OF STUDY

|  |  | Completed | Pending | Refused |
|---|---|---|---|---|
| Parents | 198 | 145 (73%) | 36 | 17 |
| Siblings | 307 | 238 (78%) | 31 | 38 |
| Children | 133 | 108 (81%) | 15 | 10 |
| Total | 638 | 491 | 82 | 65 |

To date we have found the disease to be familial in 25 instances and possibly familial in a further 12, which makes a minimum incidence of 25 per cent, or 37 per cent if the 'doubtful' cases are included (Table II).

TABLE II

FAMILIAL INCIDENCE

|  | Familial | Doubtful | Non-familial |
|---|---|---|---|
| Hypertrophic | 20 | 10 | 48 |
| Congestive | 5 | 2 | 14 |
| Total | 25 | 12 | 62 |

Further analysis of the 25 affected families showed that in the hypertrophic group a cardiomyopathy was present in 30 per cent of the parents, 40 per cent of the siblings, and 15 per cent of the children, while in the congestive group 10 per cent of the parents, 22 per cent of the siblings and 18 per cent of the children were affected, but the size of the two groups was not comparable (Table III).

Four additional points became evident during this analysis:

(*a*) The occurrence of hypertrophic and congestive cases within the same family, which has been previously reported (Nasser *et al.* 1967) but not widely accepted.

(*b*) The similarity of the sex ratio in the propositi in familial

TABLE III

ANALYSIS OF POSITIVE FAMILIES

|  | | Affected Parents | Affected Siblings | Affected Children |
|---|---|---|---|---|
| Hypertrophic | 20 | 12/40 (30%) | 26/65 (40%) | 4/28 (14%) |
| Congestive | 5 | 1/10 (10%) | 4/18 (22%) | 2/11 (18%) |

TABLE IV

SEX INCIDENCE

|  | No. | F | M | Ratio |
|---|---|---|---|---|
| Familial | 25 | 10 | 15 | 1·5 |
| Non-familial | 62 | 23 | 39 | 1·7 |

TABLE V

PREGNANCY AND CARDIOMYOPATHY

|  | No. of women | No. of pregnancies | Deaths |
|---|---|---|---|
| Familial | 16 | 43 | 0 |
| Non-familial | 9 | 18 | 0 |
| Total | 25 | 61 | 0 |

TABLE VI

AGE AT DEATH

|  | No. of cases | Average age |
|---|---|---|
| Familial | 26 | 28·9 |
| Non-familial | 18 | 41·1 |

and non-familial cases, which was 1:1·5 and 1:1·7 respectively, males being more frequently affected in both (Table IV).

(*c*) The absence of maternal deaths during pregnancy in affected women in both familial and non-familial groups, which confirmed previous observations (Turner, Oakley and Dixon 1968) (Table V).

(*d*) There was a significant difference in the age at which death occurred in the familial and non-familial cases. In the former, when all deaths due to surgery were excluded, the average age was 28·9 years, compared with 41·1 years in the latter (Table VI). The reason for this difference was not apparent.

## SUMMARY

(1) The familial incidence of idiopathic cardiomyopathy (hypertrophic and congestive) in this study was between 25 and 37 per cent.

(2) Cases with features of hypertrophic and congestive cardiomyopathy occurred in the same family.

(3) Familial cases appeared to have a worse prognosis, the average age of death being 28·9 years compared with 41·1 years in non-familial cases.

(4) There was no difference in the sex distribution of the propositi in familial and non-familial cases. Males predominated and the sex ratio was 1:1·5 and 1:1·7 respectively.

(5) There was no instance of maternal mortality in the 25 women with cardiomyopathy (familial 16, non-familial 9) during 61 pregnancies.

## REFERENCES

Evans, W. (1949) Br. Heart J. **11,** 68.

Goodwin, J. F. (1964) Br. med. J. **1,** 1527–1533; 1595–1597.

Goodwin, J. F. (1970) Lancet **1,** 731–739.

Goodwin, J. F., Gordon, H., Hollman, A. and Bishop, M. B. (1961) Br. med. J. **1,** 169–179.

Nasser, W. K., Williams, J. F., Mishkin, M. E., Childress, R. H., Helman, C., Merritt, A. D. and Genovese, P. D. (1967) Circulation **35,** 638–652.

Turner, G. M., Oakley, C. M. and Dixon, H. G. (1968) Br. med. J. **2,** 281–284.

# AN ELECTROMYOGRAPHIC STUDY IN HYPERTROPHIC OBSTRUCTIVE CARDIOMYOPATHY

I. S. Meerschwam and W. J. M. Hootsmans

*University Department of Cardiology and University
Department of Neurology, Wilhelmina-Gasthuis, Amsterdam*

In contrast to the impressive amount of knowledge about the clinical and haemodynamic characteristics of hypertrophic obstructive cardiomyopathy (HOCM) accumulated during the last decade, almost nothing is known yet about its aetiology. Several aetiological hypotheses have been formulated, but none, so far, has been confirmed. The aetiological unity of the condition has itself been questioned by some authors (Braunwald *et al.* 1964).

As soon as we began to study this condition in 1962 the concept of HOCM as a cardiac manifestation of a generalized muscular disease was considered. A link between myocardial and skeletal muscular disease is indicated by those heredofamilial muscular dystrophies (progressive muscular dystrophy, dystrophia myotonica) known to be associated with cardiomyopathy. Our attention was also drawn to this aetiological possibility by the presence of proved cases of progressive muscular dystrophy among the relatives of two of our patients.

The present study was designed to ascertain whether, in a group of patients with HOCM, indications of a generalized muscular disease could be found.

## MATERIALS AND METHODS

For the purpose of the study 40 patients were selected in whom HOCM was diagnosed after a clinical, haemodynamic and cineangiographic investigation. All patients, except one who had bacterial endocarditis, underwent right and left heart catheterization with cineangiography of the left ventricle. Right ventricular cineangiography was performed in 29 cases. The ages of the patients ranged from two to 74 years, with a median of 25 years. There were 27 males and 13 females.

The following diagnostic criteria were used for the selection of patients: (1) The presence of myocardial disease of unknown aetiology. (2) Haemodynamic evidence of outflow obstruction during ventricular systole and/or impedance of ventricular filling in diastole. (3) Cineangiographic evidence of a reduced left ventricular cavity with gross and irregular hypertrophy of the free wall and septum. Cases with a normal or dilated left ventricular cavity were excluded.

Serum enzyme activities were investigated in 31 cases. We were mainly interested in creatinine phosphokinase and aldolase activities, which may be elevated in muscular dystrophy. The upper limits of normal values in our laboratory are 1 mU/ml for creatinine phosphokinase and 8 U/ml for aldolase.

All patients were examined by a consultant neurologist. An electromyographic study was performed at least once in every patient, when at least two muscles (in most cases deltoid and quadriceps femoris) were investigated using the technique described by Buchthal (1957). A concentric needle electrode (DISA) and a two-channel Tectronics oscillograph 502 A with preamplifier 2A61 (maximum amplification 10 $\mu$V/cm) was used. The horizontal sweep velocity was 5 ms/cm and the trigger frequency of the oscilloscope beam 8 Hz. The motor unit action potentials were filmed directly from the oscilloscope screen, the film being transported vertically at a speed of 2·5 inches (6·3 cm)/s. The mean durations of 20 different groups of four identically shaped motor unit potentials were measured in every muscle investigated. From the 20 values thus obtained for each muscle, the mean duration, standard deviation, and in several cases the standard error, were calculated and compared with the normal figures given by Buchthal (1957) for the muscle tested and for age. Only deviations of 20 per cent or more from normal were considered to indicate abnormality (see Fig. 1). It is to be stressed that shortening of the duration of the potential is the main electromyographic abnormality in myogenic myopathy. The frequent occurrence of polyphasic action potentials is another indication of this disorder.

## RESULTS

In 28 cases left intraventricular outflow obstruction was demonstrated, with peak systolic pressure gradients ranging

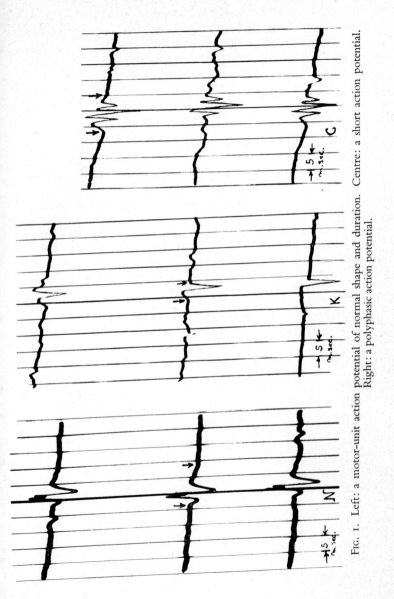

Fig. 1. Left: a motor-unit action potential of normal shape and duration. Centre: a short action potential. Right: a polyphasic action potential.

between 15 and 150 mm Hg and a median of 70 mm Hg. In 11 cases no evidence of left outflow obstruction was present either at rest or with provocation. One patient was not catheterized. Right ventricular outflow obstruction with gradients ranging between 10 and 85 mm Hg (median 16 mm Hg) was shown in ten patients. In 33 cases the left ventricular end-diastolic pressure exceeded 12 mm Hg. A complicating mitral incompetence could be demonstrated in 20 cases.

The case histories of our patients showed no complaints about muscular weakness or fatigability. In fact many of the subjects were active in sports. At routine neurological examination no clinical signs of a generalized muscular disease could be found, in any instance.

In five of the 31 patients in whom creatinine phosphokinase activity was measured, a small rise was found, ranging between 1·1 mU/ml and 1·7 mU/ml. Increased aldolase activity ranging between 9·6 U/ml and 28·6 U/ml was found in six of the 24 patients in whom this enzyme was investigated. Histological and histochemical studies of muscle biopsies obtained from three subjects showed no abnormalities.

The electromyographic study (Fig. 2) showed significant shortening of the mean potential duration ranging between 22 and 70 per cent in one or both investigated muscles in 26 of our 40 patients. In the remaining 14 no significant alteration of the mean potential duration could be demonstrated.

When the mean normal potential duration of every muscle investigated was plotted against its actual measured value (Fig. 3) most points fell in the area of potential shortening. A high incidence of polyphasic action potentials was noted in 16 cases. In 14 cases the study was repeated after intervals of between 2 and 42 months. In 13 of these cases both sets of results agreed well.

No relationship could be found between the presence of the electromyographic abnormalities and the functional class or the clinical and haemodynamic findings. A clearly positive correlation, with a correlation coefficient of 0·49, could however be demonstrated between the age of the patients and the presence or extent of electromyographic alterations, as shown in Fig. 4. Of the 15 patients under the age of 20, only four had significantly shorter action potential durations, whereas these abnormalities were present in 22 of the 25 older patients. The patients exhibiting

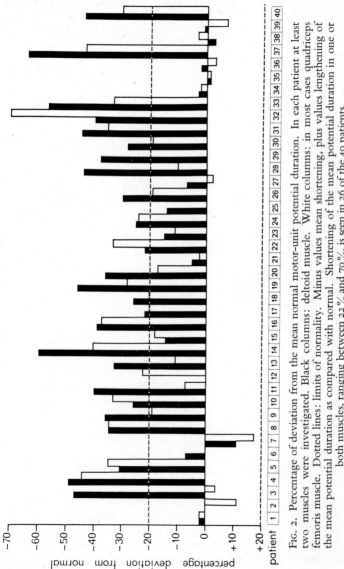

Fig. 2. Percentage of deviation from the mean normal motor-unit potential duration. In each patient at least two muscles were investigated. Black columns: in most cases quadriceps femoris muscle. White columns: deltoid muscle. Dotted lines: limits of normality. Minus values mean shortening, plus values lengthening of the mean potential duration as compared with normal. Shortening of the mean potential duration in one or both muscles, ranging between 22% and 70%, is seen in 26 of the 40 patients.

electromyographic abnormalities were significantly older (median age 31 years) than those with normal electromyograms (median age 16 years).

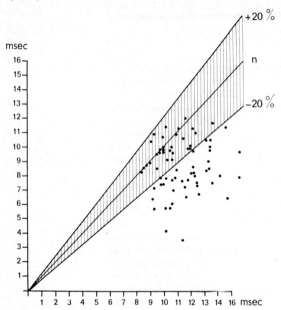

FIG. 3. The mean normal potential duration of every investigated muscle (abscissa), plotted against its actual measured value (ordinate). Most points fall in the area of potential shortening.

## DISCUSSION

The present study is an extension of an investigation of 23 patients reported in 1969 (Meerschwam 1969). To our knowledge these are the first electromyographic studies performed in patients with HOCM.

According to current views in the relevant literature (Buchthal 1957; Buchthal, Rosenfalck and Erminio 1960; Dumoulin and Aucremanne 1959; Rodriques and Oester 1956; Steinbrecher 1965), the principal abnormality of the motor unit potential in myogenic muscular disease is a lessening of its duration. The mean duration of these potentials varies from muscle to muscle and with age, and Buchthal (1957) gives the mean normal values for various muscles and different age groups. As stated above, only deviations of 20 per cent or more from normal are considered to indicate abnormality. Such shortening of the mean potential duration

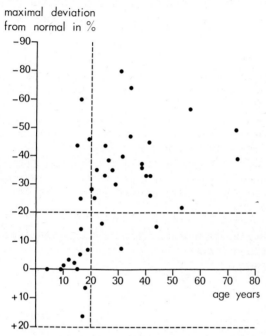

FIG. 4. Relationship between electromyographic abnormalities and age. For explanation see text.

was found in 26 of our 40 patients, i.e. in 65 per cent. In 12 of them the decrease in mean potential duration ranged between 40 per cent and 70 per cent. In addition, a high incidence of polyphasic action potentials, another feature often encountered in muscular dystrophy, was found in 16 cases.

The finding that the incidence and degree of the electromyographic abnormalities was higher in the older age group may indicate that these alterations become manifest only later in life. Our results suggest that an appreciable number of patients presenting the clinical features of HOCM have indications of a generalized asymptomatic muscular disorder. A generalized myopathy with early and serious cardiac manifestations should therefore be considered as a possible aetiological factor in this group of patients. The presence of proved cases of progressive muscular dystrophy among close relatives of two of our patients perhaps gives some additional support to our hypothesis.

## SUMMARY

An electromyographic study was performed in 40 patients with hypertrophic obstructive cardiomyopathy (HOCM). The mean duration of the motor-unit action potential was measured in several muscles and compared with normal values as given by Buchthal (1957). In 26 out of the 40 patients (i.e. 65 per cent) significant shortening of the mean potential duration was measured, suggesting the presence of generalized muscular disease in these cases. The incidence and degree of the electromyographic abnormalities increased with age. Proved cases of progressive muscular dystrophy have occurred among the relatives of two patients.

Our results suggest that in an appreciable number of patients presenting the clinical picture of HOCM, a generalized myopathy with early and serious cardiac manifestations should be considered as a possible aetiological factor.

## REFERENCES

BRAUNWALD, E., LAMBREW, C. T., ROCKOFF, S. D., ROSS, J. and MORROW, A. G. (1964) *Circulation* **30**, Suppl. IV, IV-1.

BUCHTHAL, F. (1957) *An Introduction to Electromyography*. Copenhagen: Gyldendal.

BUCHTHAL, F., ROSENFALCK, P. and ERMINIO, F. (1960) *Neurology, Minneap.* **10**, 398.

DUMOULIN, J. and AUCREMANNE, C. (1959) *Précis d'Électromyographie*. Brussels: De Visscher.

MEERSCHWAM, I. S. (1969) *Hypertrophic Obstructive Cardiomyopathy*. Amsterdam: Excerpta Medica Foundation.

RODRIQUES, A. A. and OESTER, Y. T. (1956) In *Electrodiagnosis and Electromyography*, ed. Licht, S. New Haven, Conn.: E. Licht.

STEINBRECHER, W. (1965) *Elektromyographie in Klinik und Praxis*. Stuttgart: Thieme.

# PATHOPHYSIOLOGICAL CONSIDERATIONS IN MUSCULAR SUBAORTIC STENOSIS[*]

E. Douglas Wigle, Allan G. Adelman and
Malcolm D. Silver

*Cardiovascular Unit, Toronto General Hospital, and*
*Departments of Medicine and Pathology, University of Toronto*

THE haemodynamics and pharmacodynamics of muscular subaortic stenosis have been intensively studied over the past decade and were fully discussed at the 1964 Ciba Foundation symposium on cardiomyopathies. At that time, attention was focused on left ventricular contractility, volume and afterload as being the major determinants of the severity of the outflow tract obstruction (Gorlin *et al.* 1964; Braunwald *et al.* 1964; Goodwin *et al.* 1964; Wigle 1964*a*).

In this brief discussion we should like to focus attention on the following aspects of muscular subaortic stenosis: (1) the nature of intraventricular pressure differences in man; (2) cineangiographic findings; (3) mitral regurgitation; (4) current thoughts on the nature of the outflow tract obstruction.

## THE NATURE OF INTRAVENTRICULAR PRESSURE DIFFERENCES

Although the phenomenon of catheter entrapment in myocardium was referred to in the 1964 symposium, it was Criley and co-workers (1965) who focused attention on this problem. They suggested that the intraventricular pressure difference encountered in patients with muscular subaortic stenosis might be due to this phenomenon rather than to obstruction to ventricular outflow.

In attempting to sort out the true nature of intraventricular pressure differences, several lines of approach were followed (Wigle, Auger and Marquis 1966; Ross *et al.* 1966; Wigle, Marquis and Auger 1967*a*; Wigle, Auger and Marquis 1967). As indicated in Fig. 1 (left), it was reasoned that if there was obstruction to ventricular outflow in muscular subaortic stenosis, and if the obstruction was caused by the systolic apposition of the

[*] Work supported by the Ontario Heart Foundation.

anterior mitral leaflet with the hypertrophied ventricular septum, then all intraventricular pressures proximal to the obstruction, including that just inside the mitral valve (the initial inflow tract pressure [Wigle, Auger and Marquis 1966]) should be elevated

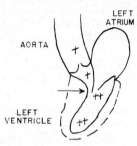

INTRAVENTRICULAR PRESSURE            INTRAVENTRICULAR PRESSURE
DIFFERENCE DUE TO                    DIFFERENCE DUE TO CATHETER
MUSCULAR SUBAORTIC STENOSIS          ENTRAPMENT IN MYOCARDIUM

FIG. 1. Left: In muscular subaortic stenosis because the obstruction to left ventricular outflow (arrow) is caused by systolic apposition of the ventricular septum and anterior leaflet of the mitral valve, the intraventricular pressure distal to the stenosis (and proximal to the aortic valve) is low (+), whereas all ventricular pressures proximal to the stenosis, including the one just inside the mitral valve (the inflow tract pressure), are elevated (+ +). Right: When an intraventricular pressure difference is recorded due to catheter entrapment from cavity obliteration, the elevated ventricular pressure is recorded only in the area of entrapment (+ +). The intraventricular systolic pressure in all other areas of the left ventricular cavity, including that in the inflow tract just inside the mitral valve, is low (+) and equal to aortic systolic pressure. The three areas of the left ventricle represented by the + 's in each of these diagrams are, from above downward, the outflow tract just below the aortic valve (subaortic region), the inflow tract just inside the mitral valve, and the left ventricular apex. (From Wigle, Auger and Marquis 1966, with permission of the editors.)

above the systolic pressure in the outflow tract and aorta. Conversely, the initial inflow tract pressure should not be elevated in cases where the elevated intraventricular pressure was due to catheter entrapment (Fig. 1, right). This hypothesis was tested extensively by ourselves and Ross and co-workers and found to

be true and a valuable means by which the obstructive intraventricular pressure gradient in muscular subaortic stenosis could
be distinguished from the artefactual intraventricular pressure
difference due to catheter entrapment. Ancillary methods of

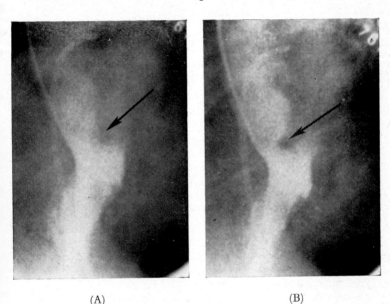

(A)                    (B)

FIG. 2. Two systolic frames from a left anterior oblique left
ventricular cineangiogram in a patient with muscular subaortic stenosis. In early systole (A) the arrow points to
the position of the anterior mitral leaflet. By mid-systole
(B) this leaflet (arrow) has encroached on the left ventricular outflow tract to cause the obstruction to outflow. At the
same time the left atrium begins to become opaque, indicating
the onset of mitral regurgitation. (From Adelman *et al.*
1969, with the permission of the editors.)

demonstrating that the catheter recording the high intraventricular pressure in muscular subaortic stenosis was in a blood-filled,
high pressure area of the left ventricle were described (Ross *et al.*
1966; Wigle, Marquis and Auger 1967*a*). It was also shown that
the left ventricular ejection time in muscular subaortic stenosis
was prolonged in proportion to the magnitude of the left ventricular-aortic pressure difference as it is in other types of aortic

stenosis. Pharmacological or surgical abolition of the pressure gradient across the outflow tract resulted in a shortened ejection time, as would be expected, with relief of an obstruction to left ventricular outflow (Wigle, Auger and Marquis 1967).

## CINEANGIOGRAPHIC STUDIES

In the past five years a number of the cineangiographic features of muscular subaortic stenosis have been elucidated (Klein, Lane and Gorlin 1965; Criley *et al.* 1965; Dinsmore, Sanders and Harthorne 1966; Rackley, Whalen and McIntosh 1966; Simon, Ross and Gault 1967; Adelman *et al.* 1969). Most of these reports have been concerned with the size and shape of the left ventricle, the appearance of the anterior mitral leaflet in relation to the site of the outflow tract obstruction and the occurrence of mitral regurgitation.

In our own studies (Adelman *et al.* 1969) there appeared to be a definite sequence of events in systole. In early systole there was an extremely rapid ejection into the aorta and the anterior mitral leaflet moved posteriorly out of the outflow tract. By mid-systole the upper ventricular septum appeared to encroach on the outflow tract anteriorly but, perhaps more importantly, the anterior leaflet of the mitral valve was seen to encroach on the posterior aspect of the outflow tract (Fig. 2). Frequently there was a radiolucent area in the outflow tract, indicating the site of obstruction to outflow caused by the systolic apposition of the anterior mitral leaflet and the ventricular septum. Mitral regurgitation became evident in mid-systole coincident with the forward motion of the anterior mitral leaflet, and was most evident in the last half of systole. The severity of the mitral regurgitation appeared to account in large measure for the degree of left ventricular emptying in the last half of systole, and hence for the small end-systolic volume of this chamber. At end-systole the two hypertrophied papillary muscles were often prominently outlined. Thus, the cineangiographic sequence of events in systole in muscular subaortic stenosis appeared to be 'eject–obstruct–leak'.

Several groups of investigators have now demonstrated that the abnormal systolic anterior movement of the anterior mitral leaflet can also be recognized by ultrasound recordings (Shah, Gramiak and Kramer 1969; Shah *et al.* 1969; Popp and Harrison 1969; Pridie and Oakley 1970).

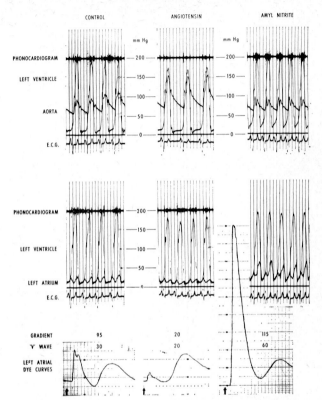

Fig. 3. Simultaneous left ventricular and aortic pressures (top) left atrial and ventricular pressures (middle) and left atrial dye curves (bottom) in a patient with muscular subaortic stenosis under control conditions (left) and following the administration of angiotensin (centre) and amyl nitrite (right). The left atrial dye curves in this and subsequent figures were performed by withdrawing left atrial blood via a trans-septal catheter during left ventricular injection of indocyanine green dye (vertical arrows) via a retrograde catheter. Dye curves are inscribed from left to right; the first upward deflection indicates the amount of mitral regurgitation, the second the recirculating dye. Angiotensin infusion decreased the severity of the subaortic stenosis as well as reducing the degree of mitral regurgitation as indicated by the dye curve and a decrease in the left atrial 'v' wave from 30 to 20 mm Hg. After amyl nitrite, the severity of the subaortic stenosis increased, as did the degree of mitral regurgitation, as indicated by the amount of early-appearing dye in the left atrial dye curve and the increase in left atrial 'v' wave from 30 to 60 mm Hg.

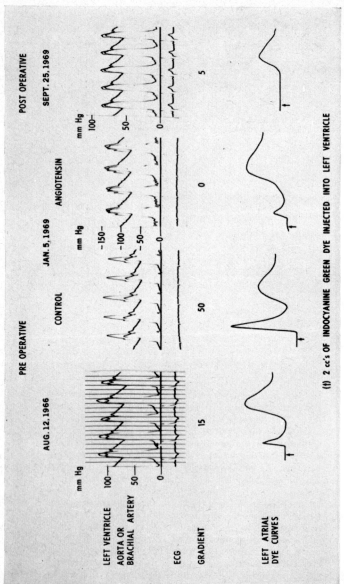

Fig. 4.

## MITRAL REGURGITATION

In addition to studying the occurrence of mitral regurgitation in muscular subaortic stenosis during cineangiography, we have also studied this important facet of the condition using indicator dilution techniques (Wigle, Marquis and Auger 1967b; Wigle et al. 1969). In these studies 2 ml of indocyanine green dye were injected into the high pressure area of the left ventricle via a retrograde catheter while blood was simultaneously and continuously withdrawn from the left atrium via a trans-septal catheter.

A total of 44 patients with muscular subaortic stenosis have been studied using these techniques. Mitral regurgitation was found in every patient in whom there was evidence of obstruction to left ventricular outflow at rest (Fig. 3).

In 20 of the 44 patients studied by dye dilution techniques we have infused angiotensin (Wigle et al. 1965) to ameliorate or abolish the outflow tract obstruction in order to assess the relation of the severity of the mitral regurgitation to the severity of the obstruction. In 16 of these 20 patients the severity of the mitral regurgitation was directly related to the severity of the obstruction to outflow (Figs. 3 and 4). When angiotensin lessened or abolished the obstruction to ventricular outflow, the mitral regurgitation

---

FIG. 4. Simultaneous left ventricular and aortic pressure recordings (top) and left atrial dye curves (bottom) pre- and postoperatively in a patient with muscular subaortic stenosis in whom the degree of mitral regurgitation was related to the severity of the outflow tract obstruction. Preoperatively between 1966 and 1969 the pressure gradient across the left ventricular outflow tract increased from 15 to 50 mm Hg and the degree of mitral regurgitation also increased, as indicated by the amount of early-appearing dye in the left atrial dye curve. During abolition by angiotensin of the outflow tract obstruction the mitral regurgitation was all but abolished, suggesting that the mitral regurgitation was related to the outflow tract obstruction and that surgical relief of the obstruction should also relieve the mitral regurgitation. After a ventriculomyotomy operation, the resting outflow tract gradient varied from 0 to 5 mm Hg and no mitral regurgitation was present, as could be predicted from the preoperative angiotensin studies.

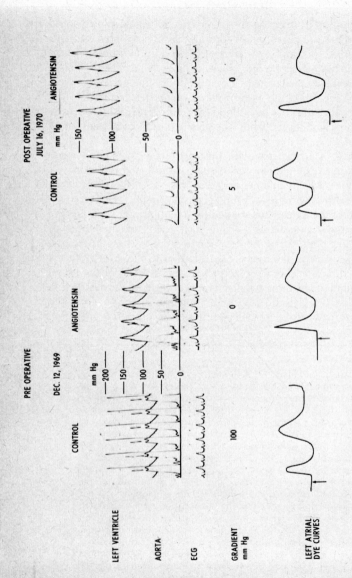

was also lessened or abolished. These preoperative studies allowed us to predict that the surgical relief of the outflow tract obstruction in these patients would also result in the abolition of the mitral regurgitation (Fig. 4).

Of the 20 patients in whom indicator dilution studies were carried out during pharmacological intervention, there were four in whom angiotensin abolished the outflow tract obstruction but failed to reduce the degree of mitral regurgitation (Fig. 5). This suggested to us that in these four patients there was an independent anatomical abnormality of the mitral valve and that the mitral regurgitation would not vanish after a successful ventriculomyotomy. Two of these four patients have subsequently come to post-mortem and both have had congenital mitral valve abnormalities (Wigle *et al.* 1969). A third patient has recently undergone surgery and although the obstruction to left ventricular outflow was relieved, the mitral regurgitation remained unchanged postoperatively (Fig. 5).

### CURRENT THOUGHTS ON THE NATURE OF THE OUTFLOW TRACT OBSTRUCTION

The fact that a muscle-splitting incision (ventriculomyotomy) in the anterior end of the hypertrophic ventricular septum in muscular subaortic stenosis abolishes the abnormal anterior movement of the anterior mitral leaflet (Shah *et al.* 1969), as well as the obstruction to left ventricular outflow and the mitral regurgitation, suggests that the myocardial abnormality in this condition is the primary fault. Since it appears that the abnormal systolic

FIG. 5. Simultaneous left ventricular and aortic pressure recordings (top) and left atrial dye curves (bottom), pre- and postoperatively, in a patient with muscular subaortic stenosis in whom the degree of mitral regurgitation was not related to the severity of the outflow tract obstruction. Abolition by angiotensin of the outflow tract obstruction preoperatively failed to decrease the degree of mitral regurgitation, suggesting that the latter was related to an anatomical abnormality of the mitral valve and was independent of the obstruction to outflow. Following surgical abolition of the outflow tract obstruction the degree of mitral regurgitation remained essentially unaltered (see text).

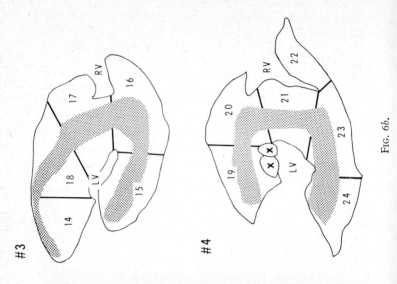

Fig. 6b.

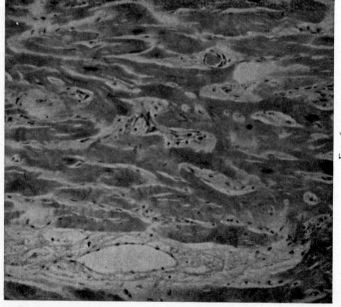

Fig. 6a.

movement of the anterior mitral leaflet can account for both the obstruction to outflow and the mitral regurgitation, the question might be asked: "How does the apparently primary myocardial fault cause this abnormal systolic movement of the anterior mitral leaflet?" Previous studies of the pathological aspects of this condition have indicated that it is characterized by gross left ventricular hypertrophy, most marked in the ventricular septum (Teare 1958; Goodwin *et al.* 1960; Braunwald *et al.* 1960; Menges, Brandenburg and Brown 1961; Wigle 1964*b*; Pearse 1964). The bizarre nature of the myocardial fibre hypertrophy has been well documented (Teare 1958; Pearse 1964). Recent studies in our laboratory have indicated that the bizarre fibre hypertrophy is centred mainly in the middle of the left ventricular wall (Fig. 6), an area normally occupied by circumferentially arranged muscle fibres (Streeter *et al.* 1969), which are largely responsible for left ventricular ejection (Lewis and Sandler 1969). Durrer and coworkers (1969) have obtained electrophysiological evidence of premature activation of the mid-left ventricular wall in muscular subaortic stenosis.

From the foregoing considerations, the following sequence of events could explain the known pathophysiological features in muscular subaortic stenosis. Accelerated activation and/or contraction of the circumferentially arranged bizarre hypertrophic myocardial fibres in the left ventricular wall could account for the

---

FIG. 6*a*. Microscopic section of the bizarre hypertrophic myocardial fibres from a patient who in life was documented as having muscular subaortic stenosis. The fibres are plump with large nuclei and course in diverse directions. Loose cellular connective tissue is seen between fibres. (Haematoxylin and eosin × ∼110.)

FIG. 6*b*. Outlines of two horizontal slices taken midway between the apex and base of the heart of a patient who in life was documented as having muscular subaortic stenosis. The numbers indicate individual full-thickness sections taken for microscopic study. L.V.=left ventricle. R.V.= right ventricle. The dark stippled areas indicate the redistribution of the bizarre myocardial fibre hypertrophy in the horizontal plane and are representative of the findings in six hearts studied in this fashion (see text).

rapid left ventricular ejection in the early non-obstructed phase of systole. This rapid ejection could draw the anterior mitral leaflet into the outflow tract by a Venturi effect, thereby producing the obstruction to ventricular outflow and the mitral regurgitation. The possibility of a Venturi effect being operative would be enhanced by the anterior leaflet being closer to the centre of the ejection path and/or by the leaflet being less taut in systole than normal. The alteration in left ventricular geometry caused by the ventricular septal hypertrophy is such that these Venturi-enhancing mechanisms could be operative. Changes in left ventricular volume, contractility and afterload, which are known to alter the severity of the subaortic stenosis and the mitral regurgitation, could do so by affecting the Venturi mechanism and hence the degree of abnormal movement in systole of the anterior mitral valve leaflet.

## SUMMARY

Pathologically, muscular subaortic stenosis is characterized by gross left ventricular hypertrophy, most evident in the ventricular septum and by microscopic evidence of bizarre myocardial fibre hypertrophy centred in the mid-left ventricular wall. Pathophysiologically it is characterized in diastole by reduced ventricular compliance and in systole by an abnormal anterior movement of the anterior mitral leaflet which accounts for the simultaneous occurrence of obstruction to left ventricular outflow (by apposition with the ventricular septum) and mitral regurgitation. In the absence of a separate anatomical abnormality of the mitral valve, the severity of the mitral regurgitation is directly related to the degree of outflow tract obstruction. Cineangiographically and ultrasonically, the anterior mitral leaflet swings into the outflow tract suddenly, in a very dynamic fashion, and does not appear to be tautened or tethered by surrounding structures. It is suggested that a Venturi effect may be responsible for the abnormal systolic movement of the anterior mitral leaflet and that this effect results from the rapid systolic ejection and altered left ventricular geometry caused by the ventricular septal hypertrophy. Changes in left ventricular volume, contractility and afterload, which are known to alter the severity of the subaortic stenosis and the mitral regurgitation, could do so by affecting the Venturi mechanism and hence the degree of abnormal systolic movement of the anterior mitral valve leaflet.

## Acknowledgements

The authors would like to acknowledge the valuable contributions of Drs P. Auger, J. Lam, Y. Marquis, M. McLoughlin and K. W. Taylor, the technical assistance of Miss J. McMeekan and staff, and of Maria Lorber and Frieda Gross, the secretarial assistance of Miss Dorothy Goodwin, the art work carried out by the Department of Art as Applied to Medicine, University of Toronto, and the photography by the Department of Medical Photography, Toronto General Hospital.

## REFERENCES

ADELMAN, A. G., McLOUGHLIN, M. J., MARQUIS, Y., AUGER, P. and WIGLE, E. D. (1969) *Am. J. Cardiol.* **24**, 689–697.

BRAUNWALD, E., LAMBREW, C. T., HARRISON, D. C. and MORROW, A. G. (1964) In *Ciba Fdn Symp. Cardiomyopathies*, pp. 172–188. London: Churchill.

BRAUNWALD, E., MORROW, A. G., CORNELL, W. P., AYGEN, M. M. and HILBISH, T. F. (1960) *Am. J. Med.* **29**, 924–945.

CRILEY, J. M., LEWIS, K. B., WHITE, R. I. and ROSS, R. S. (1965) *Circulation* **32**, 881–887.

DINSMORE, R. E., SANDERS, C. A. and HARTHORNE, J. W. (1966) *New Engl. J. Med.* **275**, 1225–1228.

DURRER, D., DAM, R. T. VAN, FREUD, G. E., MEIJLER, F. L. and ROOS, J. P. (1969) In *Electrical Activity of the Heart*, pp. 53–68, ed. Manning, G. W. and Ahuja, S. P. Springfield: Thomas.

GOODWIN, J. F., HOLLMAN, A., CLELAND, W. P. and TEARE, R. D. (1960) *Br. Heart J.* **22**, 403–414.

GOODWIN, J. F., SHAH, P. M., OAKLEY, C. M., COHEN, J., YIPINTSOI, T. and POCOCK, W. (1964) In *Ciba Fdn Symp. Cardiomyopathies*, pp. 189–213. London: Churchill.

GORLIN, R., COHEN, L. S., ELLIOTT, W. C., KLEIN, M. D. and LANE, F. J. (1964) In *Ciba Fdn Symp. Cardiomyopathies*, pp. 76–93. London: Churchill.

KLEIN, M. D., LANE, F. J. and GORLIN, R. (1965) *Am. J. Cardiol.* **15**, 773–781.

LEWIS, R. and SANDLER, H. (1969) *Circulation* **40**, Suppl. III, pp. 132.

MENGES, H. JR, BRANDENBURG, R. O. and BROWN, A. L. (1961) *Circulation* **24**, 1126–1136.

PEARSE, A. G. E. (1964) In *Ciba Fdn Symp. Cardiomyopathies*, pp. 132–164. London: Churchill.

POPP, R. L. and HARRISON, D. C. (1969) *Circulation* **40**, 905–914.

PRIDIE, R. B. and OAKLEY, C. M. (1970) *Br. Heart J.* **32**, 203–208.

RACKLEY, C. E., WHALEN, R. E. and McINTOSH, H. D. (1966) *Circulation* **34**, 579–584.

Ross, J. Jr, Braunwald, E., Gault, J. H., Mason, D. T. and Morrow, A. G. (1966) *Circulation* **34,** 558–578.

Shah, P. M., Gramiak, R., Adelman, A. G. and Wigle, E. D. (1969) *Circulation* **40,** Suppl. III, pp. 183.

Shah, P. M., Gramiak, R. and Kramer, D. H. (1969) *Circulation* **40,** 3–11.

Simon, A. L., Ross, J. Jr and Gault, J. H. (1967) *Circulation* **36,** 852–867.

Streeter, D. D., Spotnitz, H. M., Patel, D. J., Ross, J. and Sonnenblick, E. H. (1969) *Circulation Res.* **24,** 339–349.

Teare, R. D. (1958) *Br. Heart J.* **20,** 1–8.

Wigle, E. D. (1964a) In *Ciba Fdn Symp. Cardiomyopathies*, pp. 224–227. London: Churchill.

Wigle, E. D. (1964b) In *Ciba Fdn Symp. Cardiomyopathies*, pp. 49–69. London: Churchill.

Wigle, E. D., Adelman, A. G., Auger, P. and Marquis, Y. (1969) *Am. J. Cardiol.* **24,** 698–706.

Wigle, E. D., Auger, P. and Marquis, Y. (1966) *Can. med. Ass. J.* **95,** 793–797.

Wigle, E. D., Auger, P. and Marquis, Y. (1967) *Circulation* **36,** 36–44.

Wigle, E. D., David, P. R., Labrosse, C. J. and McMeekan, J. (1965) *Am. J. Cardiol.* **15,** 761–772.

Wigle, E. D., Marquis, Y. and Auger, P. (1967a) *Circulation* **35,** 1100–1117.

Wigle, E. D., Marquis, Y. and Auger, P. (1967b) *Can. med. Ass. J.* **97,** 299–301.

# AUSCULTATORY PHENOMENA IN
# HYPERTROPHIC OBSTRUCTIVE CARDIOMYOPATHY

M. Nellen, W. Beck, L. Vogelpoel and V. Schrire

*Cardiac Clinic, Department of Medicine, University of Cape Town*

The features of hypertrophic obstructive cardiomyopathy (HOCM) have been well studied over the past ten years (Braunwald, Brockenbrough and Frye 1962; Braunwald *et al.* 1964; Goodwin 1970). However, cases are still seen, as Professor Burchell mentioned here in 1964, masquerading under the diagnosis of mitral incompetence or coronary artery disease with angina. The typical patient with intraventricular obstruction shows massive asymmetrical hypertrophy of the outflow tract of the left ventricular wall. However, disorder of inflow from impairment of compliance, due to hypertrophy and muscle rigidity, may be the sole haemodynamic disorder. Thus, echocardiography (Moreyra *et al.* 1969) has shown apposition of the anterior mitral valve leaflet to the interventricular septum in diastole and reduced rapid ventricular filling slope of this leaflet. But this is not specific to HOCM. The left atrial curve shows a large 'A' wave with a small 'V' wave and a slow 'Y' descent, due to prolonged left ventricular filling. By contrast, the usual type of mitral incompetence shows a large V wave and rapid ventricular filling. The clinical picture of the disease with a mid-late systolic murmur, jerky arterial pulse, often bifid, especially in the carotid arteries, and palpable apex and left atrial beat, is well known. The cardiogram usually shows changes of left ventricular hypertrophy, yet there may be no hypertension, and this paradox should alert the clinician.

Of recent interest is Goor, Lillehei and Edwards' (1969) description of a moderate to extreme degree of 'sigmoid septum' in some hearts of people aged 51–70. They believe that this is an exaggeration of the physiological bending of the ventricular septum brought about by physiological decrease in cardiac output with ageing and shrinking of the left ventricular cavity, and that at least some of the cases published as HOCM with no intra-

78 M. NELLEN *et al.*

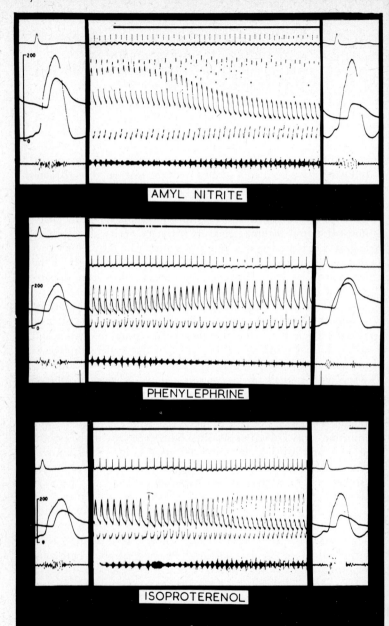

AMYL NITRITE

PHENYLEPHRINE

ISOPROTERENOL

FIG. 1.

ventricular gradient (Ewy *et al.* 1968) are probably examples of sigmoid septum with systolic murmurs. However, in a personal communication Edwards does not suggest any relationship between the two conditions.

Patients with HOCM present with dyspnoea, angina, palpitations, fatigue or syncope, but the systolic murmur in most cases draws attention to the condition, and it is on this aspect I would like to concentrate here. The murmur begins after the first heart sound, is present in about 80–90 per cent of cases and has a crescendo–decrescendo configuration with its maximum intensity to the right of mid-systole. It is best heard in the fourth or fifth left intercostal space, internal to the apex beat or confined to the apex beat or possibly radiating to the axilla. It may rarely radiate to the neck. It has a harsh low-pitched quality. Rarely it may be honking. It varies in intensity from one examination to another. Occasionally it is loud, at other times it may be soft or absent. Whilst the systolic murmur draws attention to the diagnosis, John Goodwin (1970) has described a case, followed over six years, in which the systolic murmur disappeared, the signs of obstruction changing to that of congestive failure. This is a most interesting observation in the long term, which we have also seen.

Other notable features on auscultation, in about half the cases, are the striking fourth heart sound and a softer third heart sound. In about 10–20 per cent of cases, left and right-sided delayed ventricular inflow diastolic murmurs due to inflow obstruction occur to which the occasional mitral valve thickening may contribute, and paradoxical or partial paradoxical splitting of the second heart sound occurs in about 5–10 per cent of cases. An early diastolic murmur is occasionally heard and may be due to distortion of the aortic valve ring by asymmetrical hypertrophy, and very rare early ejection clicks have been reported (Tucker *et al.* 1966), but we have not recorded this. Snellen (1964) has recorded occasional low-pitched mid-systolic sounds, preceding the onset

Fig. 1. Simultaneous left ventricular and femoral artery pressure and phonocardiogram. Top: Increase of pressure gradient and systolic murmur with inhalation of amyl nitrite. Middle: Abolition of murmur and gradient with phenyl-ephrine. Bottom: Increase of gradient and murmur with isoprenaline (isoproterenol).

or sudden increase in intensity of a high-pitched systolic murmur. Isolated obstruction within the right ventricle alone can cause a systolic murmur (Falcone, Moore and Lambert 1967). A systolic

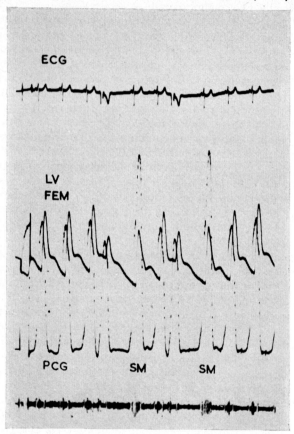

FIG. 2. Post-premature accentuation of the systolic murmur and the gradient between left ventricle (LV) and femoral artery (FEM). PCG=phonocardiogram; SM=systolic murmur.

murmur, as shown by intracardiac left ventricular phonocardiography, may rarely occur even when there is no pressure gradient in the left ventricle. However, the intensity of the systolic murmur appears, from our studies, to vary with the gradient. Thus, amyl nitrite intensifies the systolic murmur and increases the gradient; it is an excellent, and perhaps the best, means of increasing the obstructive gradient. Amyl nitrite inhalation also intensifies the systolic murmur of aortic valve stenosis, except in extremely severe cases (Vogelpoel *et al.* 1959). Phenylephrine abolishes or

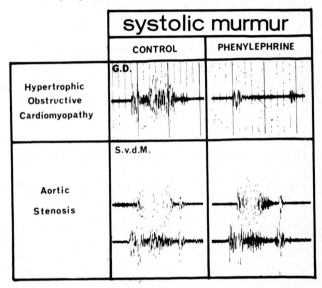

Fig. 3. Systolic murmur in mild aortic stenosis. Virtual abolition of murmur in HOCM. Slight lessening in aortic stenosis.

markedly reduces the murmur and gradient. Isoprenaline (isoproterenol) increases the gradient and the murmur (Fig. 1) (Nellen *et al.* 1967; Nellen, Gotsman and Schrire 1968; Nellen and Gotsman 1968).

In contrast to the above, amyl nitrite markedly lessens the regurgitant murmur of rheumatic valvular mitral incompetence and phenylephrine intensifies it (Vogelpoel *et al.* 1959). Thus, these drugs, by altering the internal diameter and mechanics of the obstructive hypertrophy and the valve leaflet mechanism, affect the murmur in opposite directions to its effect in pure valvular mitral incompetence. The mitral leak in HOCM is a secondary and not a primary phenomenon and pharmacological abolition of the outflow obstruction may also abolish this mitral leak. The outflow tract is extraordinarily sensitive to haemo-dynamic changes.

Again, in contrast to valvular mitral incompetence there is post-premature beat accentuation of the systolic murmur in HOCM, in keeping with the increase in gradient (Ewy *et al.* 1968),

TABLE I

THE EFFECT OF PROMPT SQUATTING IN NORMAL SUBJECTS

- Increase in effective cardiac filling pressure
- Increase in stroke output
- Small increase in peripheral arterial resistance—kinking—hydrostatic effect
- Increase in arterial mean pressure
- Increase in arterial pulse pressure
- Baroceptor response—peripheral vasodilation, bradycardia

probable factors being increased post-premature beat potentiation and a drop in peripheral resistance before this beat (Fig. 2). Murmurs of valvular mitral incompetence react with little change or may even decrease in intensity with the post-premature beat (Perloff and Harvey 1962). Murmurs secondary to fixed ventricular outflow and aortic valvular obstruction increase in intensity with the post-premature beat, behaving like HOCM in this regard (Alhomme, Welti and Facquet 1958).

In contrast to the marked lessening in intensity or disappearance of the systolic murmur in HOCM with intravenous phenyl-ephrine, the murmur of valvular aortic stenosis is hardly affected. It usually lessens only slightly, but may actually slightly intensify. This may be a useful bedside test as the two conditions may mimic each other (Fig. 3).

Prompt squatting provides a simple bedside method of acutely increasing venous return and effective filling pressure of the heart, stroke output and systemic arterial pressure and resistance (Sharpey-Schafer, 1955, 1956) (Fig. 4; Table I). It is really the converse of the Valsalva manoeuvre. We therefore studied the effect of squatting on the systolic murmur in patients with HOCM, in those with mild aortic valve stenosis and in those with mild mitral valve incompetence, as the systolic murmur in these cases may resemble that of HOCM.

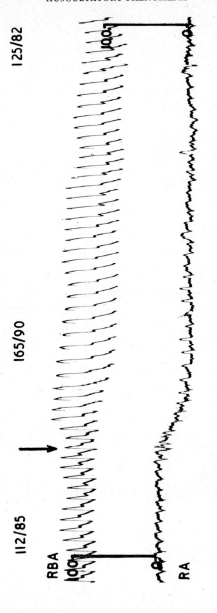

SQUATTING

FIG. 4. Right brachial pressure and right atrial pressure during the prompt squatting procedure.

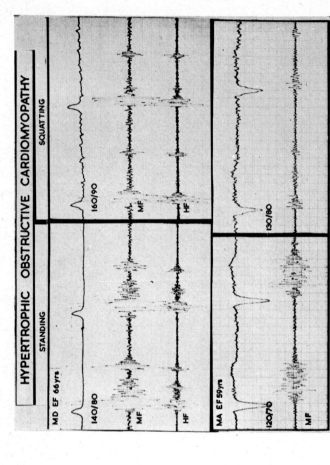

FIGS. 5 (above) and 6 (below). Virtual disappearance of systolic murmur in HOCM on prompt squatting.

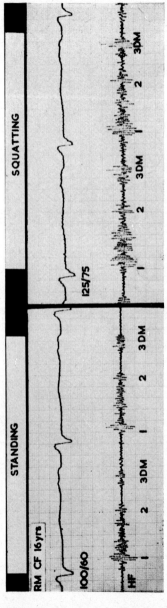

Fig. 7. Mild mitral incompetence, showing intensification of the systolic murmur.

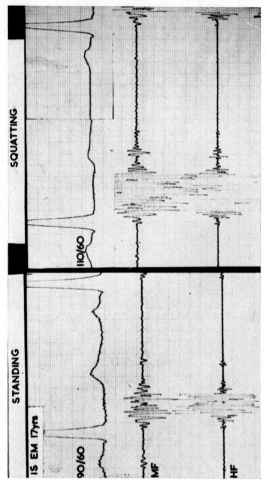

Fig. 8. Intensification of the systolic murmur in mild aortic stenosis with prompt squatting.

In HOCM we found that squatting abolished the murmur in about 30 per cent of cases and softened it significantly in a further 45 per cent. Thus, in three of every four cases, the murmur softened appreciably or was abolished (Nellen *et al.* 1967; Nellen, Gotsman and Schrire 1968; Nellen and Gotsman 1968). In the remainder it remained unchanged or softened insignificantly. In contrast, in mild valvular aortic stenosis and mild mitral incompetence the systolic murmur increased in intensity with prompt squatting (Figs. 5, 6, 7, 8).

If, on squatting, a systolic murmur markedly lessens or disappears, we have always found the diagnosis to be HOCM. So far we have not found an exception to this, and the murmur never increased in intensity.

TABLE II

RESPONSE OF SYSTOLIC MURMUR

|  | HOCM | Mitral incompetence | Aortic stenosis |
|---|---|---|---|
| Amyl nitrite | ↑ | ↓ | ↑→ |
| Phenylephrine | ↓ | ↑ | ⇄ |
| Prompt squatting | ↓→ | ↑ | ↑ |
| Post-premature beat | ↑ | ⇄ | ↑ |

The question that remains is, in which type of case does squatting fail to soften the systolic murmur appreciably?

The striking softening is not seen in very severe cases with rigid non-responsive, non-compliant chambers—just as the murmur in severe aortic stenosis with a compromised chamber function does not change with amyl nitrite inhalation. Nor is the softening seen in apprehensive patients, when presumably catecholamine production is at its highest, or when the patient is under effective doses of propranolol with a good bradycardia, the murmur being then at its lowest intensity. In addition, we suspect that where there is also an appreciable right ventricular gradient, and non-compliance of this chamber, the effect may be cancelled.

The decrease in intensity of the systolic murmur in the prompt squatting manoeuvre can be explained by the sudden increase in venous return (which also explains the intensification of a mild pulmonary valve stenosis murmur) and pulmonary outflow tract murmur. The squatting therefore must be prompt to effect this

M. NELLEN *et al.*

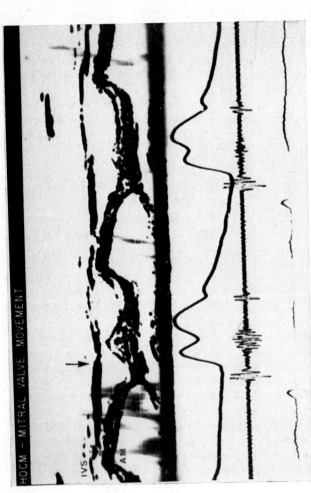

FIG. 9. Beat-to-beat variations in the amplitude of the systolic murmur, the contour of arterial pulse and the amplitude of the systolic anterior movement (SAM), in a 48-year-old woman in whom the resting pressure difference between left ventricle (LV) and brachial artery (BA) varied from 10 to 55 mm Hg, being higher during expiration. (From Shah, Gramiak and Kramer, 1969.)

sudden increase, thus leading to increased left ventricular filling and increase in diastolic volume, with, inferentially, the lessening of the gradient. In addition, the sudden raised arterial pressure, peripheral resistance and bradycardia would reduce the gradient and thus the intensity of the murmur (Table II).

The abnormal systolic anterior movement of the mitral cusp and its intimate relationship to obstruction and mitral incompetence has been convincingly demonstrated angiographically by Dinsmore, Sanders and Harthorne (1966), Simon, Ross and Gault (1967), and Wigle and his group (Adelman *et al.* 1969; Wigle *et al.* 1969), and Björk drew attention to this phenomenon at the Ciba Foundation symposium in 1964.

This sharp reopening of the aortic cusp of the mitral valve during systole, when it should normally remain in the fully closed position, has also been shown by echocardiography by Pridie (1969) and Pridie and Oakley (1970). This has been confirmed by E. Chesler (unpublished), working in our clinic. The mechanism consists of abnormal and premature papillary muscle action with consequent forward movement of the aortic valve cusp, explaining both the mitral incompetence and outflow obstruction, which are related in degree. All components augment with inhalation of amyl nitrite, which again confirms their interdependent relationship.

Shah, Gramiak and Kramer (1969) showed, very beautifully, that the onset of the systolic anterior movement coincides with the onset of the systolic murmur. Administration of methoxamine resulted in disappearance of the systolic anterior movement. In one case, this movement was temporarily related to a low frequency click (Figs. 9, 10, 11).

It would be very exciting if we could use echocardiography to show the probable change in the systolic anterior movement of the mitral leaflet on prompt squatting, but we have found this is difficult technically, and Pravin Shah concurs. It is difficult to aim the echo beam with sufficient speed and accuracy in the new posture.

### CONCLUSION

The cause and behaviour of the systolic murmur is thus unique in many respects. The mechanism of its production is not as simple as was thought when hypertrophic cardiomyopathy was first studied. It is intimately tied up with septal hypertrophy,

90 M. NELLEN *et al.*

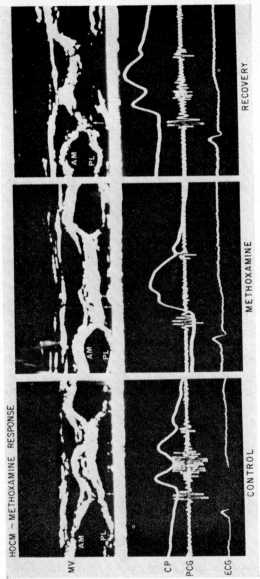

FIG. 10.

papillary muscle distortion and systolic anterior mitral valve movement, myocardial contractility, blood volume, posture, systemic blood pressure and peripheral resistance. Its main aetiological factors are intraventricular obstruction, mitral incompetence and probably turbulence within the chamber. It is a result of a complex pathogenetic aetiological situation. It sounds like mitral incompetence and mimics aortic stenosis, yet it responds in its own characteristic way to bedside manipulation of the circulation.

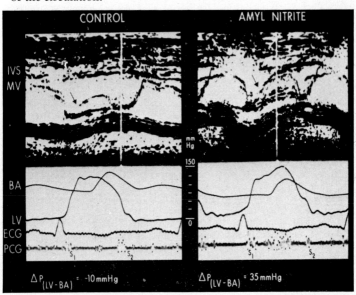

FIG. 11. Effects of amyl nitrite inhalation in a 19-year-old male who had no resting gradient across LV outflow. During peak effect of amyl nitrite the development of systolic anterior movement (SAM) is associated with an increase in the systolic murmur and the presence of systolic pressure difference between left ventricle (LV) and brachial artery (BA). (From Shah, Gramiak and Kramer 1969.)

FIG. 10. Effect of intravenous methoxamine on amplitude of systolic anterior movement and on gradient, murmur and contour of arterial pulse. (From Shah, Gramiak and Kramer 1969.)

## REFERENCES

ADELMAN, A. G., MCLOUGHLIN, M. J., MARQUIS, Y., AUGER, P. and
  WIGLE, E. D. (1969) *Am. J. Cardiol.* **24,** 689.
ALHOMME, P., WELTI, J. J. and FACQUET, J. (1958) *Archs Mal. Coeur* **51,** 493.
BJÖRK, V. D. (1964) In *Ciba Fdn Symp. Cardiomyopathies*, p. 127, p. 289.
  London: Churchill.
BRAUNWALD, E., BROCKENBROUGH, E. C. and FRYE, R. L. (1962) *Circulation*
  **26,** 166.
BRAUNWALD, E., OLDHAM, H. N., JR, ROSS, J., JR, LINHARDT, J. W., MASON,
  D. T. and FORT, L. III (1964) *Circulation* **29,** 422.
BURCHELL, H. B. (1964) In *Ciba Fdn Symp. Cardiomyopathies*, pp. 29-42.
  London: Churchill.
DINSMORE, R. E., SANDERS, C. A. and HARTHORNE, J. W. (1966) *New Engl.
  J. Med.* **275,** 1225.
EWY, G. A., MARCUS, F. I., BOHAJALIAN, O., BURKE, H. L. and ROBERTS,
  W. C. (1968) *Am. J. Cardiol.* **22,** 126.
FALCONE, D. M., MOORE, D. and LAMBERT, E. C. (1967) *Am. J. Cardiol.*
  **19,** 735.
GOODWIN, J. F. (1970) *Lancet* **1,** 731.
GOOR, D., LILLEHEI, C. W. and EDWARDS, J. E. (1969) *Am. J. Roentg.* **107,** 366.
MOREYRA, E., KLEIN, J. J., SHIMADA, H. and SEGAL, B. L. (1969) *Am. J.
  Cardiol.* **23,** 32.
NELLEN, M. and GOTSMAN, M. S. (1968) *Post-grad. med. J.* **44,** 89.
NELLEN, M., GOTSMAN, M. S. and SCHRIRE, V. (1968) *Am. Heart J.* **76,** 295.
NELLEN, M., GOTSMAN, M. S., VOGELPOEL, L., BECK, W. and SCHRIRE, V.
  (1967) *Br. med. J.* **2,** 140.
PERLOFF, J. K. and HARVEY, W. P. (1962) *Prog. cardiovasc. Dis.* **5,** 172.
PRIDIE, R. B. (1969) *Br. Heart J.* **31,** 390.
PRIDIE, R. B. and OAKLEY, C. M. (1970) *Br. Heart J.* **32,** 203.
SHAH, P., GRAMIAK, R. and KRAMER, D. A. (1969) *Circulation* **40,** 3.
SHARPEY-SCHAFER, E. P. (1955) *Br. med. J.* **1,** 693.
SHARPEY-SCHAFER, E. P. (1956) *Br. med. J.* **1,** 1072.
SIMON, A. L., ROSS, J., JR. and GAULT, J. H. (1967) *Circulation* **36,** 852.
SNELLEN, H. A. (1964) In *Ciba Fdn Symp. Cardiomyopathies*, p. 48. London:
  Churchill.
TUCKER, R. B. K., BARLOW, J. B., ZION, M. M. and GALE, G. E. (1966)
  *Proc. V Wld Congr. Cardiol.* New Delhi, p. 197.
VOGELPOEL, L., NELLEN, M., SWANEPOEL, A. and SCHRIRE, V. (1959)
  *Lancet* **2,** 810.
WIGLE, E. D., ADELMAN, A. G., AUGER, P. and MARQUIS, Y. (1969) *Am. J.
  Cardiol.* **24,** 698.

## DISCUSSION

*Grant:* Dr Emanuel, you found no genetic mechanisms which could explain the incidence of both familial and sporadic cases. One way of course would be by the occurrence of new mutations, when some of the cases are likely to appear sporadically.

*Emanuel:* I have no explanation for the sporadic cases, unless they are due to a mutation. The evidence in the familial cases suggests a dominant inheritance with variable clinical expression and variable penetrance.

*Bentall:* Have any confidence limits been established for the differences you showed?

*Emanuel:* The only significant difference in the two groups was the age of death. Familial cases had the worse prognosis.

*Bentall:* Were there any differences in the numbers of sibs and other available first-degree relatives in the two groups? The younger people, just because they are younger, may have more relatives readily available to establish that they haven't got the familial disease.

*Emanuel:* There was no significant difference in the percentage of siblings, parents and children in the two groups.

*Braunwald:* As you pointed out, we agree on almost every point and I think the sex difference is a very minor variation. Have you compared the severity of obstruction in the two groups, in which we did find a difference? And have you looked at the three points in the electrocardiogram in which we found differences: namely, the incidence of right axis deviation or indeterminate axis in the two groups, the frequency of left ventricular hypertrophy, and the frequency of intraventricular conduction defects?

*Emanuel:* No, we have not yet looked at these points.

*Burchell:* Would the emergence of symptoms in the post-partum state in a previously healthy woman exclude a case from your series?

*Emanuel:* No.

*Barratt-Boyes:* Our radiologist, Dr P. Brandt, feels that the best projection to demonstrate the abnormal movement of the anterior mitral leaflet is a left lateral one, for the cardiac apex moves downwards so that the apex of the ventricle does not overshadow the mitral area. The valve is profiled rather nearer the posterior commissure than the anterior commissure. In the normal heart the anterior mitral leaflet moves forward during diastole and there is no anterior muscular bulge of note. In the isometric contraction phase the anterior mitral leaflet closes and during systolic ejection there is very little change in its position. During isometric relaxation the leaflet is still closed.

In a patient with idiopathic hypertrophic subaortic stenosis (IHSS), with an outflow gradient above 100 mm Hg, the abnormal anterior mitral leaflet movement seen on the cineangiogram correlated very well with the gradient. During diastole the anterior muscular bulge was well seen, with the open anterior mitral leaflet approximating to it, and a wide inflow bolus into the ventricle. During isometric contraction the mitral valve closed in the normal way, then in the systolic ejection phase there was a reversed L-shaped movement of the distal one-third of the anterior leaflet towards the septum. After ejection, during the phase of isometric relaxation, this anterior movement disappeared and the leaflet returned to an almost normal position.

The catheter gradient occurs at the site of this forward anterior leaflet movement towards the hypertrophied septum and the degree of this movement correlates well with the gradient demonstrated across the outflow. In 21 patients with this condition who have been studied, only three failed to show this abnormal movement and they had no significant gradient.

The mechanism of this abnormal movement is open to debate. We imagine that it is related in some way to the absence of the normal apex-to-base systolic shortening in IHSS and to an abnormal orientation of the papillary muscles. We don't believe that the abnormal anterior mitral leaflet shelf is an essential part of this condition, but it presumably occurs as a result of these other anomalies. We imagine that this reversed L-shaped bend of the anterior leaflet occurs at the point of apposition of anterior and posterior leaflets. Mitral incompetence occurs at the time of this abnormal forward movement; it is usually a mid-systolic or late systolic event. This forward movement of the distal third of the anterior leaflet is probably exaggerated by the pressure difference across the anterior leaflet, the higher pressure in the left ventricle below this abnormal shelf tending to bring the anterior leaflet even nearer to the hypertrophied muscular septum. The backward movement of the anterior leaflet during the phase of isometric relaxation is probably due to the reversed flow of blood in the aortic outflow which normally occurs during this phase and which may be sufficient to move the leaflet back to a normal position. The isometric relaxation phase appears to be longer in these patients.

*Burchell:* Dr Meerschwam, do you attach any prognostic

significance to these abnormal action potentials in the voluntary muscle for the muscle disease *per se*?

*Meerschwam:* No. This shortening of the potential duration may be seen in very early stages of muscle dystrophy and even in people who only transmit the disease without ever being ill.

*Wigle:* We did similar electromyographic studies in 1964 and 1965 in three cases who came to surgery. The heart muscle was biopsied and examined electron microscopically, histochemically and by ordinary histology; quadriceps muscle biopsy and quadriceps and deltoid action potentials were also done. Our electromyographer did not make the very careful measurements that you did, Dr Meerschwam, but on surveying and measuring in the usual way he did not detect this shortening. We certainly agree with you that histologically there was no skeletal muscle abnormality.

You pointed out that the median age of those who did not have shortened action potential durations was 16 years, while it was 31 in those in whom they were shortened. In your serial studies did patients who initially had action potentials of normal duration subsequently demonstrate shortening?

*Meerschwam:* We repeated these studies in 14 cases after intervals of between two months and four years. Even after the longest intervals we didn't see significantly more shortening.

*Wigle:* The myopathic disorder in the heart seems to be progressive, yet your evidence that the action potential did not become progressively shortened in peripheral muscle would suggest the opposite.

*Meerschwam:* Myopathic disorder in the heart may be progressive, but it may also be stable for many decades, as we have seen in several patients. One of our patients had his first attacks of syncope at the age of 16 years; he was treated for hysteria and thereafter he was free of attacks for 25 years. When he was 41 he came into our study with recurrent syncopal attacks, angina and shortness of breath. So myocardial disease, or at least its manifestations, may be stationary over a very long period.

*Wigle:* Individual cases get quoted too often. Our own feeling from the natural history study I presented earlier is that some patients will stay stationary but the overall picture is one of progression.

*Meerschwam:* I can't agree with you. Other groups have

4*

reported many cases which showed no progression at all over a long time. Dr Braunwald has also commented about this.

*Braunwald:* Maybe we haven't waited long enough. If we all come back here six years from now, we may all agree with Dr Wigle. In some patients we saw no change in 12 years, but this doesn't mean they won't change in the future.

*Shah:* Over the last four years we have been interested in the use of pulsed ultrasound cardiography. Previous work (Gramiak, Shah and Kramer 1969) has demonstrated that when the transducer is held so as to obtain free and snapping movements of the anterior mitral leaflet, the ultrasonic 'beam' traverses the anterior wall of the right ventricle, right ventricular cavity, intraventricular septum, left ventricular outflow space and anterior leaflet of the mitral valve and left atrium posteriorly (Fig. 1). A medial and headward angulation of the transducer would enable one to obtain the recordings of the aortic root with the valve cusps.

The pattern of mitral leaflet motion in a normal subject includes a small gradual anterior motion in ventricular systole, probably related to the movement of the ring. In diastole the leaflet moves sharply forward as the valve opens and subsequent rapid filling results in posterior movement towards partial closure. Atrial systole is again associated with anterior displacement followed by posterior motion that results in valve closure at about the time of the first heart sound.

We first came across the abnormal mitral valve motion in a patient with hypertrophic obstructive cardiomyopathy (HOCM) in 1967, but failed to recognize its significance until we saw the second patient with identical findings in early 1968. It can be seen in Fig. 2 that the systolic as well as diastolic segments of anterior mitral leaflet motion are grossly abnormal. A sharp anterior movement of the leaflet begins after early ejection at about the first peak of the carotid pulse. The leaflet stays in apposition to the interventricular septum for up to 60 per cent of the ejection period. Towards end-systole the leaflet moves back to its normal position and this is associated with the second late systolic peak in the carotid pulse contour. The onset of the systolic murmur coincides with the abnormal movement. In diastole the leaflet shows little of the posterior motion seen normally during the period of rapid ventricular filling. Analysis of the aortic valve motion in the same patient revealed double

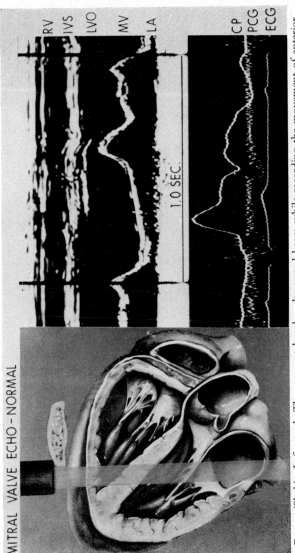

FIG. I (Shah). Left panel: The course taken by ultrasound beam while recording the movement of anterior mitral leaflet. Right panel: Recording obtained from a normal subject. RV = right ventricle, IVS = interventricular septum, LVO = left ventricular outflow space, MV = anterior leaflet of mitral valve, LA = left atrium, CP = carotid pulse, PCG = phonocardiogram, ECG = electrocardiogram.

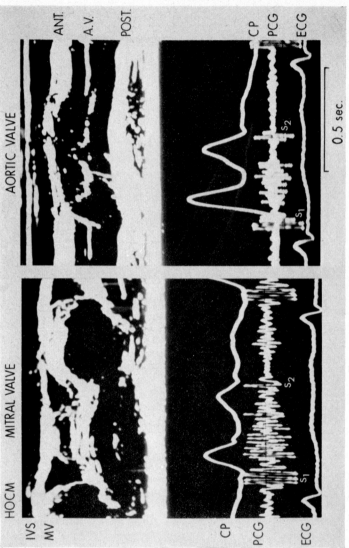

FIG. 2 (Shah). Left panel: mitral valve motion demonstrating the characteristic abnormality in systole and diastole. Right panel: Record of anterior and posterior margin of aortic root in the aortic valve (AV) cusp in between. Characteristic M-shaped configuration of the carotid pulse (CP) is involved in the aortic valve motion during

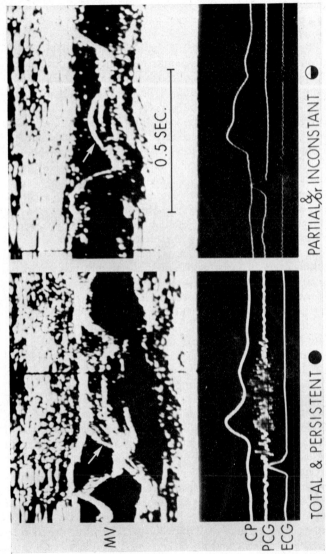

FIG. 3 (Shah). Two types of mitral valve motion abnormalities as described in the text.

systolic peaks along with the two peaks of the carotid pulse, with partial closure of the aortic cusps in mid-systole. A preliminary study of these findings has been published (Shah, Gramiak and Kramer 1968, 1969).

We subsequently collaborated with Drs Adelman and Wigle and our experience of ultrasound recordings to date extends to 50 patients. We now recognize two types of abnormalities of mitral valve motion in systole: (1) total and persistent abnormality which is present in almost every single beat recorded from the free edge of the leaflet; (2) partial and inconstant abnormality present only in occasional beats (Fig. 3). Our joint study with the Toronto group included 31 patients (Shah *et al.* 1969) in whom we analysed the echocardiographic abnormality at rest and subsequently correlated it with the left ventricular outflow gradients at rest obtained independently. Eighteen patients with persistent and total abnormality had a resting pressure gradient of 20 mm Hg or greater and often greater than 60 mm Hg. Of eight patients with no abnormality at rest seven had no resting gradient, and in one it was only 10 mm. In five patients with the partial and inconstant type of abnormality at rest, the gradients were variable (Fig. 4).

In two patients we have seen so far with cavity obliteration without true outflow obstruction, this abnormal movement was consistently absent.

We have proposed that the abnormal anterior motion results in obstruction of left ventricular outflow as well as the mitral regurgitation that invariably accompanies obstruction (Shah, Gramiak and Kramer 1968, 1969).

*O'Brien:* At Green Lane Hospital, Auckland, we have had six patients with good cineangiographic studies available for pre-operative and postoperative comparison (O'Brien, Brandt and Barratt-Boyes 1971). The abnormal mitral leaflet movement persisted in four of these, despite complete relief of the outflow gradient in three and a reduction of gradient from 124 mm Hg preoperatively to 50 mm Hg postoperatively in one. On the other hand, one patient showed complete abolition of the abnormal systolic movement and the remaining patient showed a reduction in the degree of abnormal movement. Therefore we remain uncertain about the overall changes in abnormal mitral valve movement after surgery.

*Oakley:* When the surgeon excises a bit of septum he does nothing to the mode of contraction of the ventricle or to the movement of the mitral leaflet. The gradient may go but why should the postoperative ultrasound become normal?

*Shah:* Our ultrasound studies in operated patients show

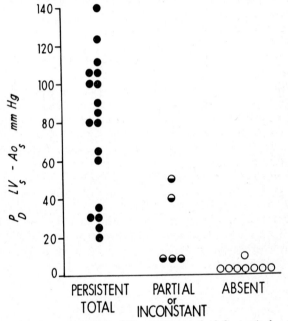

FIG. 4 (Shah). Pressure differences across the left ventricular outflow correlated with the type of mitral valve motion abnormalities noted at rest.

abolition of the abnormal mitral leaflet movement associated with relief of obstruction (Shah *et al.* 1969), as I will show later in greater detail (see p. 175).

*Wigle:* In our paper we clearly demonstrated that a ventriculomyotomy incision can abolish the abnormal systolic anterior movement of the anterior mitral leaflets as well as the obstruction to ventricular outflow and mitral regurgitation.

*Olsen:* With regard to the various abnormalities that have been described in the mitral valve, I have found at post-mortem only some elongation and thickening of the anterior mitral valve leaflet. The posterior valve leaflet also occasionally showed some thickening. This can be explained by the haemodynamic alteration. But in my experience there was no anatomical abnormality in the positioning of the mitral valve leaflets.

*Burchell:* So you believe that the anterior mitral leaflet in fact has a normal relationship to the aortic leaflets, which would not support what Dr Björk reported in 1964?

*Olsen:* Yes, in our experience. This is not to deny that in some cases an anatomical abnormality exists but I think such abnormalities are very rare.

*Braunwald:* In our experience, both surgical and at post-mortem, the anterior leaflet of the mitral valve has been thickened.

*Burchell:* Our own experience is that sometimes it is slightly thickened and sometimes it is practically normal. In a rare elderly case it may be definitely thickened and be thought to be rheumatic endocarditis.

Several people have mentioned ejection times and an explanation of how these are measured should be given. It might not mean quite the same thing in this disease as mechanical systole, ejection being possibly completed earlier than the aortic second sound. Also, in relation to end-diastolic pressure it should be stated whether the measured valve is the A wave or whether the pressure is measured at a specific time interval after the onset of QRS.

## REFERENCES

BJÖRK, V. O. (1964) In *Ciba Fdn Symp. Cardiomyopathies*, p. 127. London: Churchill.

GRAMIAK, R., SHAH, P. M. and KRAMER, D. H. (1969) *Radiology* **92,** 939.

O'BRIEN, K. P., BRANDT, P. W. T. and BARRATT-BOYES, B. G. (1971) In preparation.

SHAH, P. M., GRAMIAK, R., ADELMAN, A. and WIGLE, E. (1969) *Circulation* **40,** Suppl. III, 83.

SHAH, P. M., GRAMIAK, R. and KRAMER, D. H. (1968) *Circulation* **38,** Suppl. VI, 177.

SHAH, P. M., GRAMIAK, R. and KRAMER, D. H. (1969) *Circulation* **40,** 3.

# MANAGEMENT OF HYPERTROPHIC OBSTRUCTIVE CARDIOMYOPATHY BY BETA-BLOCKADE

M. Webb-Peploe

*Department of Medicine, Royal Postgraduate Medical School,
Hammersmith Hospital, London*

Beta-adrenergic antagonists have been widely used in the treatment of hypertrophic cardiomyopathy. There is now general agreement that intravenous administration of drugs such as pronethalol and propranolol reduces exercise and post-exercise left ventricular outflow obstruction, and prevents or reduces the increased outflow obstruction provoked by isoprenaline infusion (Braunwald *et al.* 1964). The chief benefits of long-term oral propranolol therapy appear to be relief of angina and prevention of arrhythmias (Cohen and Braunwald 1967).

Most acute studies of the effects of beta-receptor antagonism on left ventricular function in this disease have concentrated on the obstruction to left ventricular emptying, and difficulties of ventricular filling have received less attention. These patients, however, nearly all have raised left ventricular end-diastolic pressures (LVEDP) at rest, and these pressures rise still further on exercise.

We have therefore investigated the relationship between LVEDP and left ventricular work in patients with hypertrophic cardiomyopathy at rest, during mild supine leg exercise, and following injection of $2 \cdot 5$ to $5$ µg of isoprenaline into the pulmonary artery before and after intravenous administration of the cardioselective β-receptor antagonist practolol (ICI 50172, Eraldin) in doses of 20 to 40 mg.

## MATERIALS AND METHODS

In nine patients, catheters were inserted under local anaesthesia into the right median cubital vein, right brachial artery and right femoral artery, and positioned so that their tips lay in the pulmonary artery, left ventricle and aortic root, respectively.

Cardiac output (measured by indocyanine green dye dilution), and left ventricular and aortic pressures were measured at rest and during mild supine leg exercise, and also before and after infusion of isoprenaline into the pulmonary artery. Two of the patients were also atrially paced. Practolol (20 to 40 mg) was then infused into the pulmonary artery for three minutes, and the exercise and isoprenaline injection were repeated ten minutes later.

RESULTS

### Exercise

Table I shows the results obtained in six patients at rest and during exercise, before and after administration of practolol.

Before practolol, the heart rate increased from an average of 88 to 122·5 beats/min with the change from rest to exercise. Beta-adrenergic antagonism reduced but did not abolish the exercise tachycardia, the post-practolol heart rates at rest and on exercise averaging 85 and 105 beats/min respectively.

The mild level of exercise performed by these patients had no significant effect on the cardiac index. Stroke index tended to be lower on exercise than at rest, though this change was not statistically significant. Practolol did not appreciably alter these two parameters either at rest or on exercise.

Left ventricular stroke work index (LVSWI) also tended to fall with exercise, though this change did not reach statistical significance. If anything, practolol increased the level of work achieved by the ventricle both at rest and on exercise.

By far the most striking change that occurred in these patients on transition from rest to exercise was the marked rise in LVEDP. Before practolol, LVEDP rose from an average of 22 mm Hg at rest to 34 mm Hg. After practolol, the resting LVEDP averaged 18·5 mm Hg, rising to 25·5 mm Hg on exercise. The difference between pre- and post-practolol exercising levels of LVEDP was statistically significant ($P$:0·0125), and the drug was clearly exercising a beneficial effect by reducing LVEDP without depressing LVSWI.

### Isoprenaline injection

Table II shows the results obtained in all nine patients before and after isoprenaline injection, in the control state and after administration of practolol.

TABLE I

EFFECT OF PRACTOLOL ON HEART RATE, CARDIAC INDEX, STROKE INDEX, AND LEFT VENTRICULAR STROKE WORK INDEX AT REST AND ON EXERCISE IN SIX PATIENTS WITH HYPERTROPHIC CARDIOMYOPATHY

(MEAN AND S.E.M.)

| | Rest | | | Exercise | | |
|---|---|---|---|---|---|---|
| | *Before practolol* | *After practolol* | *P value* | *Before practolol* | *After practolol* | *P value* |
| Heart rate (beats/min) | 87·7±6·1 | 85·0±7·7 | 0·62 | 122·5±12·0 | 105·3±7·1 | 0·095 |
| Cardiac index (l/min m²) | 3·0±0·25 | 3·5±0·30 | 0·096 | 3·5±0·30 | 3·15±0·18 | 0·087 |
| Stroke index (m/beat m²) | 35·7±4·8 | 36·7±5·7 | 0·72 | 30·0±4·1 | 30·5±2·6 | 0·83 |
| LVSWI (g/m m²) | 47·8±7·7 | 49·7±9·2 | 0·71 | 42·6±8·4 | 43·2±6·5 | 0·85 |
| LVEDP (mm Hg) | 21·8±3·1 | 18·5±2·5 | 0·14 | 34·0±4·1 | 25·5±3·0 | 0·0125* |

★ Statistically significant at 5 per cent level.

## TABLE II

EFFECT OF PRACTOLOL ON RESPONSE OF HEART RATE AND LEFT VENTRICULAR END-DIASTOLIC
PRESSURE TO INTRAVENOUS ISOPRENALINE IN NINE PATIENTS WITH HYPERTROPHIC CARDIOMYOPATHY

| | Control | | | Isoprenaline | | |
|---|---|---|---|---|---|---|
| | Before practolol | After practolol | P value | Before practolol | After practolol | P value |
| Heart rate (beats/min) | 85·1 ± 5·1 | 83·0 ± 6·1 | 0·62 | 113·3 ± 9·9 | 96·1 ± 6·0 | 0·014* |
| LVEDP (mm Hg) | 22·6 ± 2·3 | 17·7 ± 2·6 | 0·009** | 30·0 ± 2·6 | 22·2 ± 2·1 | 0·0017** |

\* Statistically significant at 5 per cent level.
\*\* Statistically significant at 1 per cent level.

Before practolol, heart rate increased with isoprenaline from an average of 85 to 113 beats/min. After practolol this increase was from 83 to 96 beats/min. This reduction in isoprenaline tachycardia as a result of β-receptor antagonism was statistically significant ($P$: 0·014).

After injection of isoprenaline, LVEDP rose from an average of 22·5 to 30 mm Hg. After practolol, the control and post-isoprenaline LVEDP figures were 17 and 22 mm Hg. Both in the control state and after isoprenaline injection practolol thus produced a highly significant reduction in LVEDP in these nine patients ($P < 0·01$).

*Atrial pacing*

Two patients were atrially paced in addition to being given isoprenaline. In both cases the LVEDP fell with pacing to heart rates well in excess of those obtained with doses of isoprenaline sufficient to cause a marked rise in LVEDP.

### DISCUSSION

Previous workers have also noted that in hypertrophic cardiomyopathy LVEDP is often high at rest, rising still further during exercise and after administration of isoprenaline. They concluded that ". . . left ventricular function was abnormal at rest with displacement of the function curve to the right, while during exercise left ventricular function became still more abnormal" (Braunwald *et al.* 1964). Our results at first sight appear to support this conclusion, which implies that in hypertrophic cardiomyopathy stimulation of cardiac β-receptors causes a decrease in myocardial contractility, while β-receptor antagonism results in an increase in contractility. This is, of course, the exact reverse of the situation in both the normal heart and every other kind of heart disease.

Such a conclusion is, however, based on the assumption that end-diastolic pressure is an index of myocardial fibre length, and that pressure changes accurately reflect changes in volume, i.e. that left ventricular diastolic compliance does not change. One cause of an apparent decrease in diastolic compliance is extreme tachycardia (Mitchell, Linden and Sarnoff 1960), but the results of atrial pacing in our patients demonstrated that the rise in LVEDP with exercise and isoprenaline was not a rate effect due to incom-

plete ventricular relaxation as a result of diastole being shortened
by the tachycardia.

It is generally agreed that under constant conditions it is
probably safe to assume that left ventricular diastolic distensibility
does not change. Is such an assumption valid, however, firstly
under conditions of β-receptor stimulation and antagonism, and
secondly where the heart muscle is grossly abnormal?

We are at present trying to answer this question by measuring
left ventricular end-diastolic volume (LVEDV) as well as LVEDP
and LVSWI before and after administration of practolol.

## RELATIONSHIP BETWEEN LVEDV, LVEDP, AND LVSWI: PRELIMINARY RESULTS

LVEDV is calculated from simultaneously inscribed indocyanine green dye and thermal ventricular wash-out curves (Holt 1966),
and also from single-plane cineangiograms (Greene *et al.* 1967).
So far eight patients have been examined. Two patients under-
going coronary angiography for suspected ischaemic heart
disease were found to have normal coronary arteries and good
left ventricular function (referred to as normals in Figs. 1 and 2).
A third patient did have atheroma of right and circumflex
coronary arteries, but good ventricular function. Two patients
had congestive cardiomyopathy. Three patients had hypertrophic
cardiomyopathy; in two the disease was severe, but in the third
it was only mild. None of these patients had mitral regurgitation
either clinically or on the left ventricular cineangiograms.

The two 'normal' patients and the patient with ischaemic heart
disease all had normal or near-normal values for LVSWI and
LVEDP (Fig. 1). Administration of practolol caused a slight increase in both LVSWI and LVEDV, with no significant change in
LVEDP.

Of the two patients with congestive cardiomyopathy, one had
a normal LVSWI, while in the other it was depressed. LVEDP
was 17 and 15 mm Hg respectively. Both, as expected, had
grossly dilated left ventricles. In both cases practolol caused a
further increase in LVEDV accompanied by little change in
LVSWI and a rise in LVEDP (barely significant in one case, but
from 17 to 24 mm Hg in the other).

The three patients with hypertrophic cardiomyopathy all had
lower than normal values for LVSWI. This was particularly

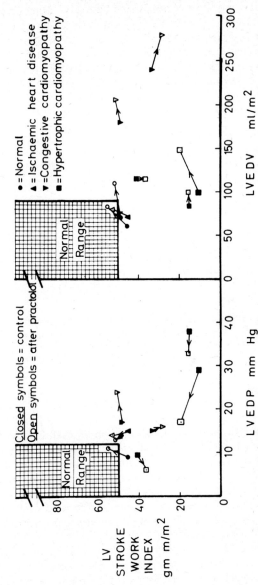

FIG. I. Effect of practolol on the relationship between left ventricular stroke work index (ordinates) and (in left panel) left ventricular end-diastolic pressure (abscissa); in the right panel is shown the relationship between LVSWI and left ventricular end-diastolic volume (abscissa). Results are shown for eight patients: 2 with normal LV function, I with ischaemic heart disease and good LV function, 2 with congestive cardiomyopathy, and 3 with hypertrophic cardiomyopathy.

marked in the two severe cases who also had gross elevation of the LVEDP. LVEDV was normal or only slightly increased in all three patients. Practolol caused an increase in LVEDV in the two severely affected cases, accompanied by a slight increase in LVSWI. In the mild case LVEDV did not change, and LVSWI fell slightly. In all three cases practolol caused a significant fall in LVEDP.

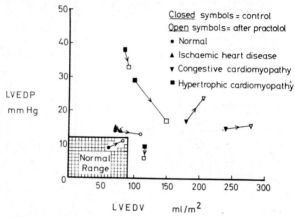

FIG. 2. Effect of practolol on relationship between left ventricular end-diastolic pressure (ordinate) and left ventricular end-diastolic volume (abscissa) in the same 8 patients as in Fig. 1. Note that in the patients without hypertrophic cardiomyopathy practolol causes an increase in LVEDV with no change or a rise in LVEDP, whereas in the patients with hypertrophic cardiomyopathy there is a rise in LVEDV accompanied by a fall in LVEDP.

Comparison of the effects of practolol on LVEDP and LVEDV (Fig. 2) showed that in all the patients who did not have hypertrophic cardiomyopathy, β-receptor antagonism caused an increase in LVEDV accompanied by no change or an increase in LVEDP. By contrast, in the patients with hypertrophic cardiomyopathy practolol caused no change (in the mild case) or an increase in LVEDV accompanied by a significant decrease in LVEDP in all three cases.

Increase in LVEDV accompanied by no change or a rise in LVEDP (as observed after practolol in our patients who did not suffer from hypertrophic cardiomyopathy) might be explained by a shift from one point to another on the same left ventricular diastolic distensibility curve, and does not permit one to conclude that a change in distensibility has occurred. Where an increase in LVEDV is accompanied by a decrease in LVEDP (practolol had this effect in the patients with hypertrophic cardiomyopathy), it is possible to state with certainty that an increase in diastolic compliance has occurred.

These preliminary results thus suggest that in hypertrophic cardiomyopathy, antagonism of the cardiac β-receptors causes an increase in left ventricular compliance. Practolol, by making the ventricle more distensible, and thus lowering LVEDP while maintaining or increasing myocardial fibre length and stroke work, should be of considerable benefit to these patients with their grossly hypertrophied and 'stiff' ventricles.

## SUMMARY

Nine patients with hypertrophic cardiomyopathy have been studied at cardiac catheterization before and after intravenous administration of practolol (ICI 50172, Eraldin), a cardioselective β-receptor antagonist. The results suggest that practolol may be of benefit in the treatment of hypertrophic cardiomyopathy, since, following its acute administration, the same cardiac work is achieved at a lower left ventricular end-diastolic pressure (LVEDP).

Left ventricular end-diastolic volume (LVEDV) is now being measured as well as LVEDP and left ventricular stroke work index (LVSWI). Preliminary results in eight patients indicate that in those who do not have hypertrophic cardiomyopathy practolol causes an increase in LVEDV accompanied by no change or a rise in LVEDP. In patients with hypertrophic cardiomyopathy, practolol causes an increase in LVEDV accompanied by a fall in LVEDP. The beneficial effects of practolol in hypertrophic cardiomyopathy may therefore be due to an increase in left ventricular diastolic distensibility.

## REFERENCES

BRAUNWALD, E., LAMBREW, C. T., ROCKOFF, S. D., ROSS, J. JR and MORROW, A. G. (1964) *Circulation* **30**, IV, IV–1.
COHEN, L. S. and BRAUNWALD, E. (1967) *Circulation* **35**, 847.

GREENE, D. G., CARLISLE, R., GRANT, C. and BUNNELL, I. L. (1967) *Circulation* **35,** 61.

HOLT, J. P. (1966) *Am. J. Cardiol.* **18,** 208.

MITCHELL, J. H., LINDEN, R. J. and SARNOFF, S. J. (1960) *Circulation Res.* **8,** 1100.

# BETA-ADRENERGIC BLOCKADE IN HYPERTROPHIC CARDIOMYOPATHY WITH EMPHASIS ON EXERCISE STUDIES

ARNI KRISTINSSON

*University Hospital, Reykjavik, Iceland*

DRUGS which block beta-receptors have been used extensively in the treatment of hypertrophic cardiomyopathy. There is still some controversy over their benefit. This may be due to the difficulty of assessing the effects of drugs on a disease with a generally very protracted course and of obscure nature. Various methods have been employed in this assessment, as shown in Table I. The results reported during the past six years will now be briefly summarized.

## SYMPTOMS

It is not always realized that β-blockers exhibit a competitive antagonism. The degree of blockade therefore is dosage-dependent (Dollery, Paterson and Conolly 1969). This may

### TABLE I

METHODS OF ASSESSING THE EFFECTS OF β-BLOCKING DRUGS IN PATIENTS WITH HYPERTROPHIC CARDIOMYOPATHY

(1) Clinical studies, symptoms and signs
(2) Haemodynamic measurements
(3) Provocation with drugs
(4) Angiographic measurements
(5) Ultrasound techniques
(6) Exercise testing

partly account for the differences in symptomatic relief reported for long-term oral treatment with propranolol (Table II): syncope and angina are most frequently relieved but effort dyspnoea is not so consistently improved. Sloman (1967) and Cohen and Braunwald (1968) maintain that congestive heart failure is a contraindication for treatment with propranolol, while Flamm,

113

Harrison and Hancock (1968) consider persistent outflow obstruction an indication for surgical rather than medical therapy.

The effects of propranolol on clinical signs have been variable and on the whole not rewarding.

TABLE II

THE EFFECTS OF LONG-TERM ORAL TREATMENT WITH PROPRANOLOL ON SYMPTOMS IN HYPERTROPHIC CARDIOMYOPATHY

| Authors | No. of patients treated | No. improved | Dose (mg) |
|---|---|---|---|
| Wigle (1965) | 3 | 1 | 120 |
| Scheu, Bollinger and Wirz (1966) | 2 | 2 | 120 |
| Cherian et al. (1966) | 13 | 10 | |
| Sloman (1967) | 5 | 4 (1 sustained) | 120 |
| Rosenblum et al. (1967) | 10 | 7 | |
| Bliss, Moffat and Gantt (1967) | 4 | 3 (0 sustained) | 160–480 |
| Cohen and Braunwald (1968) | 8 | 5 (3 sustained) | 160–480 |
| Flamm, Harrison and Hancock (1968) | 11 | 10 | 120–160 |
| Bernstein and Mitchell (1969) | 6 | 3 | 40–160 |
| Parker (1969) | 4 | 2 | |
| Swan et al. (1971) | 47 | 9 | 60–240 |
| Total | 113 | 56 | |

HAEMODYNAMICS, PROVOCATION WITH DRUGS AND ANGIOGRAPHY

The haemodynamic effects and the response to provocation with drugs after pronethalol at rest have been thoroughly discussed by Braunwald and co-workers (1964a) and Goodwin and co-workers (1964). The experience with propranolol has been similar and the results are summarized in Table III. Flamm, Harrison and Hancock (1968) found that propranolol abolished the left ventricular aortic pressure gradient in patients with latent and labile pressure gradients and reduced this gradient substantially in those patients with persistently high gradients. Bernstein and Mitchell (1969) report a reduction of the outflow tract gradient in three of 18 patients given 5 mg propranolol intravenously.

Left ventricular volume studies have been performed in patients with hypertrophic cardiomyopathy (Grant et al. 1968; Hugenholtz *et al.* 1970), but no direct measurements are available on the effects of propranolol on left ventricular volume.

TABLE III

HAEMODYNAMIC EFFECTS OF PROPRANOLOL (150 MG/KG) ON THE RESTING PATIENT

|  | Cherian et al. (1966) | Flamm, Harrison and Hancock (1968) |
|---|---|---|
| Heart rate | Reduced | Reduced |
| Cardiac output |  | Reduced |
| Stroke volume |  | Reduced |
| LVSP | Slight reduction | Reduced |
| LVEDP | Unchanged | Unchanged |
| LV-aortic gradient, resting | Slight reduction | Often reduced |
|   Isoprenaline increase | Abolished | Abolished |
|   Amyl nitrite increase |  | Unchanged |
|   Post-ectopic increase | Variable | Unchanged |
|   Valsalva increase | No change | Abolished in some |

LVSP: Left ventricular systolic pressure.
LVEDP: Left ventricular end-diastolic pressure.

### ULTRASOUND

The ultrasound technique has recently been employed in studying the movement of the mitral valve in patients with hypertrophic cardiomyopathy (Shah, Gramiak and Kramer 1969; Pridie and Oakley 1970). Popp and Harrison (1969) have reported abolition of abnormal mitral valve movement after acute and chronic administration of propranolol.

### EXERCISE TESTING

Most exercise studies on patients with hypertrophic cardiomyopathy have been designed to investigate the haemodynamic abnormality (Braunwald *et al.* 1964*a*, *b*; Flamm, Harrison and Hancock 1968). Supine leg exercises were used in those studies, but Mason, Braunwald and Ross (1966) have shown that body position influences the outflow tract gradient in patients with hypertrophic cardiomyopathy. The cardiovascular, respiratory and metabolic responses of six patients to erect submaximal exercise were therefore studied before and after acute and chronic administration of propranolol (Edwards *et al.* 1970). Their physical working capacity at a heart rate of 170 beats per minute before propranolol was less than in normal subjects, due to the high heart rate on exercise in the patients (Table IV). Heart rate rose less on exercise after the administration of propranolol (Fig. 1). This was more pronounced after three months' oral treatment,

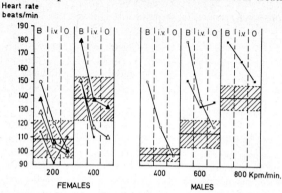

FIG. 1. Changes in heart rate on exercise before (B) and after intravenous (i.v.) and oral (O) propranolol compared with normal responses (hatched areas). Connected symbols represent individual patients exercising at work loads of 200, 400, 600 or 800 kp/m min (200, 400, 600 or 800 × 9·807 N/m min).

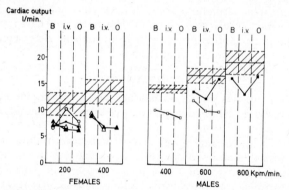

FIG. 2. Changes in cardiac output on exercise. Symbols as in Fig. 1.

implying a higher degree of β-blockade. High heart rate on exercise in cardiac disease is often associated with a low cardiac output and this was the case in these patients (Fig. 2). The augmen-

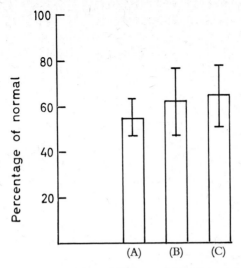

FIG. 3.  Stroke volume at highest work load for each patient, with the average value for all 6 patients expressed as a percentage of normal.  (A) indicates values obtained before, (B) after intravenous and (C) after oral propranolol.

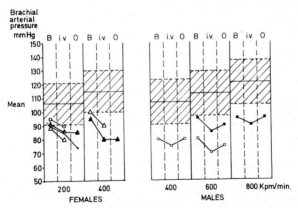

FIG. 4.  Changes in brachial artery mean pressure on exercise.
Symbols as in Fig. 1.
(Figs. 1, 2 and 4 from Edwards *et al.* 1970, by permission of the Editor, *British Heart Journal.*)

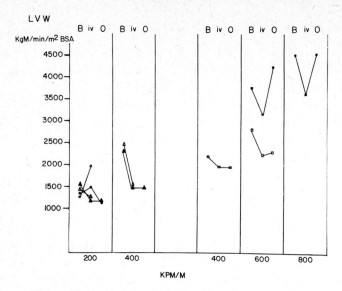

FIG. 5. Changes in left ventricular work (LVW) on exercise.
Symbols as in Fig. 1. LVW is calculated as cardiac output ×
brachial artery mean pressure × 1·36 (sp. gr. Hg) × 1·05 (sp. gr.
whole blood) divided by body surface area × 100.

## TABLE IV

PHYSICAL WORKING CAPACITY AT A HEART RATE OF 170 BEATS PER MINUTE
(P.W.C.$_{170}$) BEFORE ADMINISTRATION OF PROPRANOLOL

| Patient | Sex | Age | P.W.C.$_{170}$ (kp/m min) |
|---|---|---|---|
| A.L. | F | 21 | 375 |
| L.C. | F | 25 | 340 |
| S.K. | F | 22 | 440 |
| J.S. | F | 20 | 385 |
| Female normal subjects | | | 635 ± S.D. 105 (Pope, Higgs and Clode, unpublished data) |
| B.N. | M | 21 | 760 |
| C.B. | M | 33 | 780 |
| Male normal subjects | | | 1037 ± S.D. 224 (Edwards et al. 1969) |

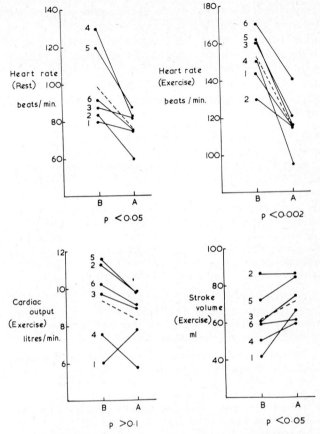

FIG. 6. Effects of practolol on heart rate at rest (upper left), heart rate during exercise (upper right), cardiac output during exercise (lower right) and stroke volume during exercise (lower right). B = before, A = after practolol.

tation of cardiac output was less on exercise in these patients than in normal controls, and propranolol had little effect.

Calculated stroke volume averaged only 55 per cent of normal values in the control studies, rising slightly after propranolol (Fig. 3). Brachial artery pressure was low on exercise and fell after propranolol. The fall was more pronounced in the systolic

5

pressure but is best shown by the electronically integrated mean pressure (Fig. 4). Left ventricular work calculated as a product of cardiac output and mean arterial pressure is shown in Fig. 5. This was slightly reduced after propranolol, as expected. Ventilation tended to be high on exercise and the effects of propranolol were small and inconsistent. Arterial lactate increased excessively on exercise before drug administration and was equally raised after propranolol.

TABLE V

THE RESULTS OF ADMINISTERING PROPRANOLOL AND PRACTOLOL DURING EXERCISE TO PATIENTS WITH HYPERTROPHIC CARDIOMYOPATHY

|  | *Propranolol* | *Practolol* |
|---|---|---|
| High heart rate | Lowered | Lowered |
| Low cardiac output | Not increased | Not increased |
| Low stroke volume | Slight increase | Increased |
| Systemic blood pressure | Lowered | Lowered |
| Left ventricular work | Reduced | ? |
| High ventilation | Little effect | Little effect |
| High blood lactate | Little effect | Little effect |

TABLE VI

ADVANTAGES OF EXERCISE TESTING IN PATIENTS WITH HYPERTROPHIC CARDIOMYOPATHY

(1) Observations made in upright posture cover exertion range of activities encountered in daily life
(2) Abnormalities not obvious at rest may become apparent
(3) Objective measure of effort intolerance
(4) Not traumatic, easily repeatable at intervals and hence the effects of drugs affecting exercise tolerance can be followed

An exercise study was performed before and after acutely administered practolol in six patients, all of whom had been taking propranolol for 6–22 months (Croxson et al. 1971). The results were similar, but calculated stroke volume seems to be higher after practolol (Fig. 6). The two studies are not strictly comparable since different methods were used in measuring cardiac output.

The results of the two exercise studies are summarized in Table V. It must be emphasized that these results can be obtained with ease and the study by Croxson and co-workers (1971) was even performed without any blood sampling, using the graphical analysis of $CO_2$ transport as described by McHardy, Jones and Campbell (1967). The advantages of exercise testing are numerous, as tabulated in Table VI.

## CONCLUSION

Sonnenblick, Ross and Braunwald (1968) have emphasized the important determinants of myocardial oxygen consumption

### TABLE VII

THE EFFECTS OF PROPRANOLOL AND PRACTOLOL ON FACTORS INFLUENCING MYOCARDIAL OXYGEN UPTAKE DURING EXERCISE

|  | Propranolol | Practolol |
|---|---|---|
| Intramyocardial tension: |  |  |
| LVEDP | Unchanged | Lowered |
| LV volume | Increased? | Unchanged |
| LV mass | Unchanged | Unchanged |
| Heart rate | Reduced | Reduced |
| Contractile state ($V_{max}$) | Reduced | Reduced |
| Basal metabolism | Unchanged | Unchanged |
| External work (muscle shortening × load) | ? | ? |

LVEDP: left ventricular end-diastolic pressure.
LV: left ventricular.
$V_{max}$: maximal velocity of myocardial contraction.

### TABLE VIII

BENEFITS OF PROPRANOLOL AND PRACTOLOL IN PATIENTS WITH HYPERTROPHIC CARDIOMYOPATHY

(1) Block catecholamine stimulation and hence lower oxygen consumption during exercise; reduce angina
(2) Prevent rise in left ventricular filling pressure on exercise; reduce dyspnoea (practolol)
(3) Reduce outflow tract gradient (propranolol)
(4) Prevent sudden death by preventing arrythmias?
(5) Arrest disease process?

($M\dot{V}O_2$). There are various gaps in our knowledge of the effects of propranolol and practolol on these. Both drugs reduce $M\dot{V}O_2$ during exercise by reducing heart rate and contractile state by blocking catecholamine stimulation (Table VII). Cohen and Braunwald (1968) have suggested that left ventricular volume is increased after propranolol and thereby intramyocardial tension and $M\dot{V}O_2$, but Webb-Peploe and co-workers (1971) have shown that left ventricular end-diastolic pressure (LVEDP) is lowered after practolol without increasing left ventricular volume, with a consequent reduction in $M\dot{V}O_2$. The effects of β-blockers on external work are not clear.

Because they reduce $M\dot{V}O_2$, clinical symptoms and the outflow tract gradient, a case is made for a trial use of propranolol or practolol in hypertrophic cardiomyopathy (Table VIII). Practolol may be the drug of choice since it reduces LVEDP, in contrast to propranolol, and thereby reduces $M\dot{V}O_2$ further. On the other hand, practolol seems to be less effective in reducing the outflow tract gradient. It is tempting to think that these drugs will prevent sudden death through their anti-arrythmic properties. Some patients have died suddenly while on treatment with propranolol, but as mentioned earlier the blockade is dosage-dependent and this question must remain in doubt. Due to the protracted natural history of the disease later experience will tell whether β-blockers will arrest the disease process, as suggested by some authors.

Further research is indicated on the effects of catecholamines on the disease. More pressure and volume studies after β-blockade would also be rewarding. Finally it is necessary to follow up patients carefully, both those who are taking β-blocking drugs and those who are not, and here exercise tests will play an important part.

### SUMMARY

Results obtained with the β-blocking drug propranolol in patients with hypertrophic cardiomyopathy are reviewed. Two exercise studies before and after propranolol and practolol are described. It is concluded that propranolol and practolol reduce myocardial oxygen consumption, clinical symptoms and the outflow tract gradient, but to different degrees, and therefore a therapeutic trial of these drugs is warranted. Further research is urged into the actions of β-blocking drugs on patients with hypertrophic cardiomyopathy, and the lines along which serial assessments of drug effects may be made in the future have been indicated.

### REFERENCES

BERNSTEIN, L. and MITCHELL, A. S. (1969) *Israel J. med. Sci.* **5**, 803–805.

BLISS, H. A., MOFFAT, J. E. and GANTT, C. L. (1967) *Circulation* **35–36,** Suppl. II, 72.

BRAUNWALD, E., LAMBREW, C. T., HARRISON, D. C. and MORROW, A. G. (1964a) In *Ciba Fdn Symp. Cardiomyopathies*, pp. 172–188. London: Churchill.

BRAUNWALD, E., LAMBREW, C. T., ROCKOFF, S. D., ROSS, J. JR and MORROW, A. G. (1964b) *Circulation* **30,** Suppl. IV, 93–101.

CHERIAN, G., BROCKINGTON, I. F., SHAH, P. M., OAKLEY, C. M. and GOODWIN, J. F. (1966) *Br. med. J.* **1,** 895–898.

COHEN, L. S. and BRAUNWALD, E. (1968) *Prog. cardiovasc. Dis.* **11,** 211–221.

CROXSON, R., JONES, G., McFADDEN, R. and WARRELL, D. A. (1971) In preparation.

DOLLERY, C. T., PATERSON, J. W. and CONOLLY, M. E. (1969) *Clin. Pharmac. Ther.* **10,** 765–799.

EDWARDS, R. H. T., JONES, N. L., OPPENHEIMER, E. A., HUGHES, R. L. and KNILL-JONES, R. P. (1969) *Q. Jl exp. Physiol.* **54,** 394–403.

EDWARDS, R. H. T., KRISTINSSON, A., WARRELL, D. A. and GOODWIN, J. F. (1970) *Br. Heart J.* **32,** 219–225.

FLAMM, M. D., HARRISON, D. C. and HANCOCK, E. W. (1968) *Circulation* **38,** 846–858.

GOODWIN, J. F., SHAH, P. M., OAKLEY, C. M., COHEN, J., YIPINTSOI, T. and POCOCK, W. (1964) In *Ciba Fdn Symp. Cardiomyopathies*, pp. 189–213. London: Churchill.

GRANT, C., RAPHAEL, M. J., STEINER, R. E. and GOODWIN, J. F. (1968) *Cardiovasc. Res.* **2,** 346–355.

HUGENHOLTZ, P. G., ELLISON, R. C., URSCHEL, C. W., MIRSKY, I. and SONNENBLICK, E. H. (1970) *Circulation* **41,** 191–202.

McHARDY, G. J. R., JONES, N. L. and CAMPBELL, E. J. M. (1967) *Clin. Sci.* **32,** 289–298.

MASON, D. T., BRAUNWALD, E. and ROSS, J. JR (1966) *Circulation* **33,** 374–382.

PARKER, B. M. (1969) *Ann. intern. Med.* **70,** 903–911.

POPE, H. M., HIGGS, B. E. and CLODE, M. Unpublished observations.

POPP, R. L. and HARRISON, D. C. (1969) *Circulation* **40,** 905–914.

PRIDIE, R. B. and OAKLEY, C. M. (1970) *Br. Heart J.* **32,** 203–208.

ROSENBLUM, R., FRIEDEN, J., DELMAN, A. J. and BERKOWITZ, W. D. (1967) *Circulation* **35–36,** Suppl. II, 226.

SCHEU, H., BOLLINGER, A. and WIRZ, P. (1966) *Cardiologia* **49,** Suppl. 2, 43–48.

SHAH, P. M., GRAMIAK, R. and KRAMER, D. H. (1969) *Circulation* **40,** 3–11.

SLOMAN, G. (1967) *Br. Heart J.* **29,** 783–787.

SONNENBLICK, E. H., ROSS, J. JR and BRAUNWALD, E. (1968) *Am. J. Cardiol.* **22,** 328–336.

SWAN, D., BELL, B., OAKLEY, C. M. and GOODWIN, J. F. (1971) *Br. Heart J.* in press

WEBB-PEPLOE, M. M., CROXSON, R. S., OAKLEY, C. M. and GOODWIN, J. F. (1971) To be published.

WIGLE, E. D. (1965) *Fedn Proc. Fedn Am. Socs exp. Biol.* **24,** 1279–1286.

## DISCUSSION

*Barratt-Boyes:* How accurate is your measurement of left ventricular end-diastolic volume in this sort of heart with gross trabeculation?

*Webb-Peploe:* In absolute terms it is probably not terribly accurate. With the thermodilution dye method trabeculation will not necessarily make much difference, but with the angiographic method we do run into trouble with queer shapes. But these two methods of measuring end-diastolic volume invariably agreed in the direction in which the volume shifted. In absolute measurements the discrepancy averaged 35 per cent, with the dye method giving us larger values than the angiographic method, which is slightly better than reported in the literature (Bartle and Sanmarco 1966).

*Braunwald:* The results are extremely interesting but I am reluctant to accept them yet. I have very little confidence in the indicator dilution method for measuring ventricular volume with any degree of precision; there is substantial evidence in the literature to justify this doubt. Again, using single-plane cineangiography for measuring volume in a ventricle as distorted as that in IHSS is extremely hazardous. We have been very interested in the problem of ventricular volume in these patients, but have been unable to calculate it, even from biplane cineangiograms. The conclusion that one can change the compliance of the myocardium *in vivo* is a far-reaching one which opposes many other observations. I don't say that it is impossible for a drug to alter ventricular compliance acutely, but the onus to prove it lies on the investigator who claims that it happens, and the techniques involved should be scrupulous. There have been many studies on isolated cardiac muscle in which one can control and measure both muscle length and resting tension with an enormous amount of precision. In such studies even large doses of catecholamines or of β-blocking agents have not altered myocardial distensibility. Similar observations have been made on intact hearts in experimental animals in which the measurements are still far more accurate than those just described in patients, where the measurements of ventricular volume are of uncertain validity.

*Oakley:* The distortion of the left ventricular cavity seen in end-systole is virtually absent in end-diastole, when the cavity shape approximates to the 'ellipse' seen in the normal ventricle. The main interest of Michael Webb-Peploe's findings lay in the reduction of rest and exercise end-diastolic pressures after practolol had been given. If no change in compliance had occurred then the end-diastolic volume must have actually got *smaller* after practolol. It is inconceivable to me that the β-blocking drugs would cause the volume, which is already normal rather than large, to get even smaller. How could they bring this about except by a gross loss in stroke volume—and we know that stroke volume was maintained? These findings therefore seem likely to be right, irrespective of the question of the accuracy of the volume findings, because of the extreme improbability of β blockade being followed by further shrinkage of these small end-diastolic volumes.

*Wigle:* What were the relative changes in cardiac output before and after practolol?

*Webb-Peploe:* There was no change.

*Wigle:* One of your cases showed no change in volume, another showed minimal change and in one case only was there a large increase in volume.

*Webb-Peploe:* All three cases showed a significant fall in left ventricular end-diastolic pressure.

TABLE I (SHAH)

RESULTS OF THE STUDY ON THE SYSTOLIC ABNORMALITY OF THE MITRAL VALVE MOTION AT REST

| Abnormal mitral leaflet motion | Untreated group | Propranolol therapy | Post-surgery group |
|---|---|---|---|
| Persistent and total | 14 | 16 | 1 |
| Partial and inconstant | 2 | 2 | 2 |
| Absent | 2 | 1 | 11 |
| Total studies (51 in 37 patients) | 18 | 19 | 14 |

*Shah:* We have examined the effects of propranolol administered either intravenously or orally on the ultrasound detection of the abnormal mitral valve motion described earlier (p. 96). This study is once again a joint effort between the Rochester and Toronto groups of investigators. Fifty-one total studies were carried out in 37 patients (Shah *et al.* 1969). Eighteen studies were performed while the patients were on no treatment, 19 while they were receiving daily oral propranolol therapy in a dose of 60–300 mg/day and 14 in patients who had undergone ventriculo-myotomy (Table I).

No significant difference in the severity of ultrasound abnormality was detected between the untreated group and those on propranolol therapy. Twelve patients were studied twice at intervals of five months with and without treatment. No significant difference in the ultrasound abnormalities was noted. Similarly, intravenous administration of propranolol in a dose of $0 \cdot 15$ mg/kg body weight in five patients had no significant effect on ultrasound abnormality. In none of these patients was a major drop in outflow pressure gradient noted despite some decrease in heart rate.

*Goodwin:* After long-term treatment (about three years) with propranolol of 40 patients with hypertrophic cardiomyopathy we found it was extraordinarily difficult to get any hard data which would convince us that we had done anything at all except relieve angina (Goodwin 1970). Certainly dyspnoea, which is very relevant in view of Webb-Peploe's results, did not seem to be improved much in these patients. We don't know the long-term results with practolol yet. The dramatic reductions in end-diastolic pressure, which Dr Oakley quite rightly emphasized, perhaps encourage us to think that practolol will be better than propranolol. We have had patients who have died suddenly while taking propranolol, although some of them were on small doses.

*Oakley:* Assessing these patients simply by their symptoms is very difficult. This came out clearly in the exercise testing studies by Dr Kristinsson and Dr Richard Edwards (Edwards *et al.* 1970). These patients often have a profound disability but it develops so slowly that they are unaware of it. It was amazing to find that patients in the N.Y.H.A. classification I or II were sometimes unable to exercise beyond 200 kp/m min ($200 \times 9 \cdot 807$ N/m min). I suppose the same may apply in reverse if they are benefited by drug treatment.

*Goodwin:* I wasn't suggesting that we had not necessarily helped the patients with propranolol, but that it was very difficult to *prove* that we had.

*Wigle:* In our experience, patients with outflow tract obstruction at rest have a gradient, a sharp anterior movement of the anterior mitral leaflet and also mitral regurgitation. Patients with latent outflow tract obstruction have no gradient, no mitral regurgitation and no ultrasound abnormality of the anterior mitral leaflet, but all three abnormalities can be provoked with appropriate pharmacological agents. Propranolol can abolish not only the gradient stimulated by isoproterenol (isoprenaline) but also that stimulated by amyl nitrite. This perhaps is worth noting.

Of our 21 patients treated with propranolol, ten were Class II in the N.Y.H.A. classification before therapy and seven of these improved to Class I. Two of these seven had latent outflow tract obstruction and the other five have only been followed for an average of 15 months (versus 27 months follow-up in patients initially in Class III–IV). Two remained in Class II and one deteriorated to Class III–IV. Of the ten patients who were Class III–IV to begin with, two improved to Class I and again these had latent outflow tract obstruction. These were the two most dramatic results that we had. One of these patients had angina and syncope for five years and the other for 15 years, and they are both back at work now full-time. Two Class III–IV patients improved initially to Class II on propranolol but the improvement has not been maintained. At the end of the follow-up period, four patients were still in Class III–IV; they had shown initial improvement, then deteriorated again, but they became even worse if we took them off propranolol. We feel that there is some evidence that propranolol can help patients with resting obstruction to outflow, but that the progression of the myocardial disorder overtakes this help. Like Professor Goodwin, we had two patients who died while on propranolol therapy. Five patients who deteriorated while on propranolol therapy have subsequently undergone surgery successfully. The four patients with latent outflow tract obstruction benefited most from propranolol therapy. The benefit of propranolol therapy to patients with resting obstruction has not been well maintained when they have been followed for over two years. Progression of the primary myocardial disease appears to overcome the benefits of propranolol therapy.

*Burchell:* Dr Webb-Peploe, did you observe any difference in the diastolic pressure slopes, before the onset of atrial systole, in the patients on practolol?

*Webb-Peploe:* We saw a decrease in the pre-A wave level of

5*

end-diastolic pressure after practolol. We haven't analysed the slopes.

*Burchell:* What was the atrial pressure generated by the atrial contraction during electronic pacing as compared with the values in exercise?

*Webb-Peploe:* The post-A-wave pressure came down with pacing.

*Braunwald:* How did you calculate ventricular work?

*Webb-Peploe:* We measured the left ventricular mean systolic pressure by planimetering by hand the left ventricular pressure trace during the ejection phase.

*Braunwald:* Did practolol reduce the left ventricular systolic pressure in the basal state?

*Webb-Peploe:* No.

*Braunwald:* Did it change the gradient?

*Webb-Peploe:* Yes, it did in most of these patients. We measured the peak systolic gradient at rest before and after practolol in these nine patients. In the group without appreciable obstruction practolol didn't alter the gradient, but in a substantial number of patients with obstruction we recorded a higher gradient at rest after practolol than before. This is in contrast to a patient to whom we gave propranolol, in whom we would expect the reverse to happen and in whom the resting gradient did, in fact, fall. On exercise this effect of practolol was rather less marked; only in two out of six patients did we see an increase in the outflow tract obstruction.

*Goodwin:* This highlights the two points of view: on the one hand the importance of outflow obstruction and on the other the importance of inflow restriction. We seem to have two different effects with these two β-blocking drugs. One perhaps has its main effect on reducing outflow gradients and the other on reducing end-diastolic pressure. Which is the more important?

*Oakley:* There is no doubt in my mind that it is the end-diastolic pressure which is more important. Our patients who have died had the highest end-diastolic pressures (as measured, but with all the limitations of 'spot' measurements) and developed atrial fibrillation, embolism, pulmonary oedema and right ventricular failure. Patients with outflow tract obstruction but with lower end-diastolic pressures did not die either suddenly or gradually. Dr Webb-Peploe's emphasis on the exercise end-diastolic pressure is very important because the end-diastolic pressure is often not particularly raised at rest but it rises rapidly on modest effort and any drug which can keep it from rising may help to slow down the progression of the disorder, although I agree that deterioration is likely in most patients eventually.

*Burchell:* But isn't this the end stage you are predominantly studying?

*Oakley:* We probably do not get the patients until the myocardial disorder is well advanced, but they may not have any detectable abnormality earlier.

*Shah:* I have some reservations about the actual measurement of end-diastolic pressures following the peak of the A wave. This is subject to variations based on P-R interval relationships, height of the A kick, etc. Since β-adrenergic blockade is likely to have some effect on the force of atrial contraction and the height of the A wave, I wonder whether the observed changes in end-diastolic pressures are explained on that basis. It would be helpful to know what happened to the mean left atrial pressures in these patients after administration of practolol.

*Webb-Peploe:* We didn't measure mean left atrial pressure because we had a catheter in the left ventricle and another catheter in the pulmonary artery. The pressure throughout the whole of diastole was lower in the left ventricle after practolol; it wasn't just a phenomenon of reducing the A kick. The difference in the effects of practolol and propranolol on the outflow gradient makes one wonder how important the peripheral effect of propranolol is in abolishing the gradient. Propranolol (but not practolol) blocks peripheral dilator β receptors, leading to peripheral vasoconstriction, and this may account for the difference that we are seeing between these two drugs in their effect on left ventricular outflow obstruction.

*Goodwin:* On the question of prognosis and end-diastolic pressure, in our patients who died suddenly we could really find no consistent feature. The nearest to any sort of consistency was elevation of the end-diastolic pressure.

*Burchell:* I am still resistant to the idea of grouping all the patients with idiopathic left ventricular enlargement as cases of obstructive cardiomyopathy. I see many individuals who have hypertrophied hearts and some of them have myocardial fibrosis.

Certainly when the end-diastolic pressure is very high we recognize it may be an unfavourable sign, but I am not sure that these non-obstructed cases have evolved from the type of problem which I have thought of as an obstructive cardiomyopathy to begin with. The incidence of emboli in Dr Oakley's series is particularly interesting. Did any of these patients show endocardial fibrosis which more or less mimicked the focal endocardial sclerosis so characteristically associated with hypertrophy and peripheral emboli? Did any of them look like 'adult-type endocardial sclerosis' to the pathologist?

*Goodwin:* I would say no, but in one or two there may have been local areas of endocardial thickening, although certainly not generalized.

*Olsen:* Yes, that is right, but only in those cases where no dilatation has taken place.

*Goodwin:* Doesn't anyone who has had 'congestive heart failure' tend to develop endocardial thickening?

*Olsen:* Yes. If the heart dilates, the endocardium becomes thickened and fibrosed, and this can lead to fibrin deposition and therefore thrombus formation. It is a non-specific reaction which occurs whenever dilation develops, even if severe hypertrophy had previously existed.

*Goodwin:* In this group of conditions the ventricle doesn't usually dilate; extensive endocardial thickening would not be expected to occur and in fact it doesn't, does it?

*Olsen:* It does not if the ventricles do not dilate.

*Oakley:* Embolism has been associated with atrial fibrillation in every patient except one, and in that patient it may well have been paroxysmal for all we know.

*Burchell:* I agree with Dr Olsen; Dr J. E. Edwards and I have also emphasized that hypertrophy in the left ventricle can lead to endocardial thickening. It has been our contention that some of the individuals who had this diagnosis of a focal type of endocardial sclerosis probably had a hypertrophied ventricle to begin with. Did these individuals who had emboli also have atrial fibrillation or did the emboli occur independently of atrial fibrillation?

*Oakley:* It is important to emphasize that (1) we saw some patients who had passed through a 'classical' phase of outflow tract obstruction before going into a phase of congestive failure, and (2) these patients when they were in congestive failure had normal end-diastolic volumes in the left ventricle. This is why we now include other patients whom we have not seen in the earlier and maybe obstructive phases of the disease and no longer either segregate them as examples of 'idiopathic hypertrophy' or confuse them with patients who have had dilated left ventricles from day one of their disease, so-called 'congestive cardio-myopathy'.

## REFERENCES

BARTLE, S. H. and SANMARCO, M. E. (1966) *Am. J. Cardiol.* **18,** 235.

EDWARDS, R. H. T., KRISTINSSON, A., WARRELL, D. A. and GOODWIN, J. F. (1970) *Br. Heart J.* **32,** 219–225.

GOODWIN, J. F. (1970) In *Cardiovascular Beta-adrenergic Responses*. UCLA Forum in Medical Science, vol. 13, p. 161. Los Angeles: University of California Press.

SHAH, P. M., GRAMIAK, R., ADELMAN, A. and WIGLE, E. (1969) *Circulation* **40,** Suppl. III, 83.

# THE SURGICAL ANATOMY OF THE HEART AND CONCEPTS OF SURGICAL TREATMENT

H. H. Bentall

*Department of Surgery, Royal Postgraduate Medical School,
Hammersmith Hospital, London*

I PROPOSE to consider very briefly the embryology and anatomy of the musculature of the ventricles for I am convinced that it will assist our understanding both of the nature of hypertrophic cardiomyopathy and of the surgical implications.

By about the 23rd day of intrauterine life the heart is a straight tube having an aortic sac, a bulbus cordis, a ventricle and a right and a left atrium which are joined to the ventricle by a short atrioventricular canal. This simple tube during the next three days bends upon itself completely, so as to bring the atria up to the level of the bulbus cordis, from the lower part of which the primitive right ventricle will arise. The primitive left ventricle arises from the original ventricular portion of the heart tube. During the next few days septation occurs and there is further twisting along the long axis so that the right ventricle comes to lie slightly in front of the left ventricle. These changes are well advanced by five weeks and virtually complete at the end of six weeks. From this brief description it is apparent that the musculature of the right ventricle arises largely from the original myo-epicardium surrounding the bulbus cordis, and that of the left ventricle from the myo-epicardium surrounding the original ventricle. Secondary attachments occur but in general the left ventricular muscle fibres have a different origin and attachment from the right ventricular fibres.

One of the earliest anatomical and physiological descriptions of the musculature of the heart is that of Borelli in 1680 and 1681, and a great deal of his description is still valid today. Many anatomists, over the last 300 years, have contributed to our understanding but in my view the most comprehensive description was that given by Franklin P. Mall from Johns Hopkins University in 1911, following a brilliant piece of original work by one of his students, John Bruce McCallum, in 1900. Most of the illustrations which follow are after Mall (1911).

After removal of the epicardium bundles of fibres are visible to the naked eye. These bundles are not entirely free but are anastomosing with each other constantly, producing the gross appearance of a syncytium, although functionally and microscopically

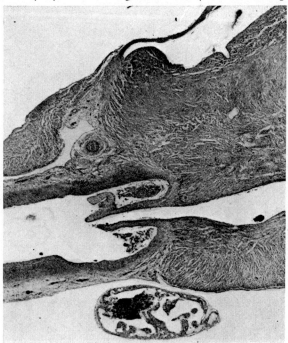

FIG. 1. Sagittal section of heart of 60 mm embryo showing pulmonary valve and right ventricular cavity. The musculature attachments to the fibrous ring of the mitral valve are clearly seen. (× 28.)

this is not a true syncytium. The bundles are in general parallel to each other, but change direction as they penetrate the wall of the heart so that those on the inside lie at right angles to those under the epicardium. In general, the superficial fibres are transverse over the right ventricle and vertical over the left ventricle. These superficial fibres arise from the tendinous rings surrounding the atrioventricular valves, and from the aorta and pulmonary artery and the tendon between them (Fig. 1). Those fibres arising from the left side of the left atrioventricular ring, the left side of the aorta and from the conus sweep down to enter the posterior horn of the vortex and thence into the septum, while those from the right

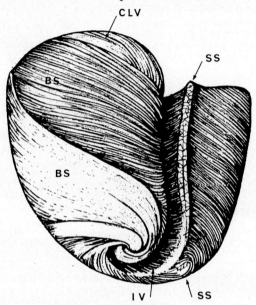

FIG. 2. Drawing of the posterior aspect of the dissected heart (after Mall). The superficial sinospiral band (SS) has been divided. BS: Superficial bulbospiral muscle and deep bulbospiral muscle; CLV: circular muscle of left venous ostium; IV: interventricular bands.

atrioventricular ring posteriorly sweep round to the front to form the anterior horn of the great vortex, ultimately entering the papillary muscle of the left ventricle.

There are thus recognized two distinct muscle groups, and it is to these that Mall gave names which have stood the test of time. Those arising from the conus and from the aorta, anatomically the aortic bulb, descend in a spiral direction to the vortex and then enter the septum. These he called the bulbospiral bundle. The other group taking origin in the venous (sinus) end of the embry-

onic heart takes a complementary course to the apex to the back
of the heart and he named this the sinospiral bundle. Each of these
groups may be further subdivided into superficial and deep
components. Fig. 2 is a view of the back of the ventricles prepared
after the method of McCallum in which the superficial sinospiral

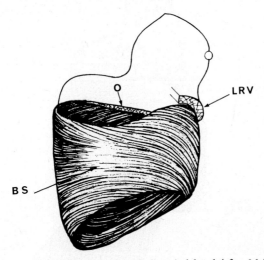

FIG. 3. Drawing of the deep bulbospiral band (after Mall)
seen from the septal aspect. O: origin of fibres of this band
from left side; LRV: longitudinal muscle of right ventricle.

muscle has been partly removed back to the posterior longitudinal sulcus and the right and left ventricles have been partly
separated from each other along a natural plane of cleavage. The
deep bulbospiral band is seen entering the septum above the superficial bulbospiral band. It will be seen that the superficial bulbospiral muscle is the most vertical and enters the apex of the heart
at the vortex, while the deep bulbospiral band is more transverse
and enters the septum appreciably higher. A much smaller, nearly
circular band of the same group of fibres is the circular muscle
band of the left venous ostium and is all that remains of the original
circular muscle of the primitive heart tube. Fig. 3 is the septal
aspect of the left ventricle showing only the deep bulbospiral band
with the outline of the aorta superimposed. The right coronary
ostium is seen. Fig. 4 shows the anterior aspect of the heart with

the superficial bulbospiral band reflected, and the deep bulbospiral band removed entirely. It will be seen that the superficial fibres, after they have entered the vortex, ascend in the septum and then

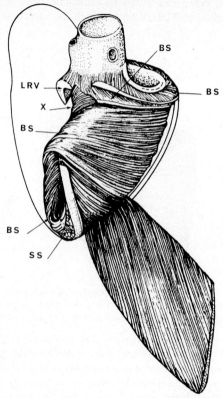

Fig. 4. Drawing of anterior aspect of heart (after Mall). The superficial bulbospiral muscle (BS) has been reflected and the deep bulbospiral muscle removed except for its origin (BS). The circular course of the superficial fibres (BS) ends at X.

sweep on the inside once again internally to the deep bulbospiral fibres, blending with them on the posterior aspect of the heart after having encircled the ventricle one-and-a-half times. Many authors have described such a figure-of-eight course for the superficial bulbospiral muscle but such a course may not be invariable.

Fig. 5 shows the deep bulbospiral band which was removed from the previous specimen, superimposed upon the same general outline and seen from the same view. The cut ends marked 'O' represent the line of attachment to the aorta and anterior parts of the atrioventricular ring from the previous illustration.

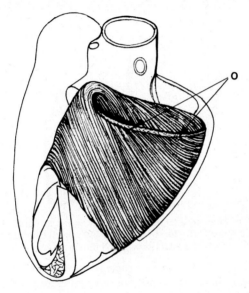

FIG. 5. The deep bulbospiral band which was removed from the heart in Fig. 4. O is the origin of the fibres shown in Fig. 3.

The work of Flett (1927) is anatomically largely confirmatory of that of Mall and the other authors. His diagram shown here in Fig. 6 depicts the upper fibres of the deep bulbospiral muscle rather more obliquely than most authors. However, he is interesting in his discussion on the function of the deep bulbospiral muscle. He quotes Lewis (1917) as stating definitely that the fibres of the base contract later than the fibres nearer to the apex, and both he and Flett considered that the deep bulbospiral band was responsible for the final ejection of the ventricular contents into the aorta. However, another function he ascribes to this muscle, as does Campbell (1921), is that it assists the support of the aortic valve against the elastic recoil of the aortic wall at the end of systole. This is in keeping with Borelli's idea of the formation of an 'intumescence internally' and, he states, seems to fulfil all the requirements as regards timing. While this may be true and is in accord with modern thinking, there is no developmental or anatomical evidence for the deep bulbospiral muscle either in whole or in part being functionally a separate entity, and any

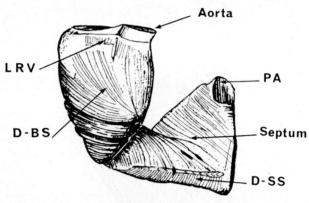

FIG. 6. Drawing after Flett showing the ventricles unrolled by McCallum's method. D–BS: Deep bulbospiral band; D–SS: deep sinospiral fibres; PA: Pulmonary artery.

additional function to that of the expulsion of blood may only be brought about by its position and differences of timing of contraction.

If we regard this disease, as I believe we must, as a primary muscle disease rather than a functional incapacity, then any obstructive element in the left ventricular outflow tract will be due to the extent to which the deep bulbospiral muscle and the adjacent part of the septum are hypertrophied. This hypertrophy may by its bulk alone, or by a combination of bulk and unbalanced contraction, produce left ventricular outflow obstruction. It seems to me that it is only in these patients that a surgical attack would be reasonable. I do not think there is the slightest evidence for any primary role of the deep bulbospiral muscle in the aetiology of this disease and I think that the use of the term 'hypertrophy' in this connexion should be abandoned. In those patients in whom ventricular filling is at fault or in those whose obstruction is inconstant (and this probably constitutes the bulk of patients), it is hard to see how surgery can offer anything. Whether the route of approach should be trans-aortic, trans-ventricular or trans-septal through the right ventricle, or a combination of any of these, will be discussed by other speakers.

## REFERENCES

BORELLI, G. A. (1680) *De Motu Animalium Pars Prima*, Tab. 16 & 17. Romae.
BORELLI, G. A. (1681) *De Motu Animalium Pars Altera*, p. 108. Romae.
CAMPBELL, H. (1921) *Br. med. J.* **1,** 542.
FLETT, R. L. (1927) *J. Anat.* **62,** 439–475.
McCALLUM, J. B. (1900) *Johns Hopkins Hosp. Bull.* **9,** 307–335.
MALL, F. P. (1911) *Am. J. Anat.* **11,** 211
LEWIS, T. (1917) *Proc. R. Soc.* **89,** 560.

# IDIOPATHIC HYPERTROPHIC SUBAORTIC STENOSIS:
## A Current Assessment of the Results of Operative Treatment

Andrew G. Morrow, Stephen E. Epstein, Bradley M. Rodgers
and Eugene Braunwald

*Clinic of Surgery and Cardiology Branch, National Heart and Lung Institute,
National Institutes of Health, Bethesda, Maryland*

At the Ciba Foundation Symposium on Cardiomyopathies in
1964, the early experiences at the National Heart Institute with
the operative treatment of idiopathic hypertrophic subaortic
stenosis (IHSS) were described (Morrow, Lambrew and Braunwald 1964). At that time the diagnosis of IHSS had been established in 64 patients, and in ten of these operation had been carried
out. IHSS has now (September 1970) been recognized in more
than 200 patients studied at the Institute, and operations designed
to relieve obstruction to left ventricular outflow have been
performed in a total of 43 patients. A current evaluation of the
clinical and haemodynamic results of operation in these 43 patients
is presented in the report which follows.

### PREOPERATIVE FINDINGS

The 43 patients, at the time of operation, ranged in age from
10 to 64 years; 27 were men or boys, 16 were women. In one-
fourth of the entire group the disease was known to be familial.

### TABLE I

INCIDENCE OF SPECIFIC SYMPTOMS DESCRIBED PREOPERATIVELY
BY 43 PATIENTS WITH IHSS

| Symptom | No. of patients |
|---|---|
| Angina pectoris | 33 |
| Dyspnoea with effort | 31 |
| Orthopnoea | 27 |
| Syncope | 26 |
| Paroxysmal nocturnal dyspnoea | 23 |
| Right heart failure | 22 |
| Paroxysmal supraventricular arrhythmia | 9 |
| Angina + syncope + congestive failure | 11 |

The patients presented the clinical, radiographic and electro-cardiographic findings characteristic of IHSS. All patients were severely symptomatic; 19 were in functional Class IV (New York Heart Association), 23 in Class III, and one in Class II. The incidence of specific symptoms is shown in Table I. In recent years almost all patients operated upon have first been treated with, and found to be unimproved by, the administration of propranolol or other beta-adrenergic blocking agents.

Every patient was studied by means of right and left heart catheterization on one or more occasions. A systolic pressure gradient between the left ventricle and the aorta or a systemic artery was present under resting basal conditions in 36 patients; these gradients ranged from 6 to 175 mm Hg (average 77 mm Hg). In the seven patients without pressure gradients at rest, large gradients became evident in post-extrasystolic beats and following one or more provocative interventions. The left ventricular end-diastolic pressure was abnormally elevated (> 12 mm Hg) in 31 of the 43 patients (range 14 to 32 mm Hg, average 22).

### OPERATIVE METHODS AND RESULTS OF OPERATION

The operation performed has previously been described in detail (Morrow *et al.* 1968; Morrow 1969). During cardio-pulmonary bypass and mild (30°C) general hypothermia, a vertical aortotomy is made, and the aortic valve is retracted. Two parallel incisions, about 1 cm apart, are made through and over the hypertrophic ridge or mound of muscle in the intraventricular septum and lateral free wall of the left ventricle. The deep muscle layers between the incisions are then split by digital pressure to a depth of approximately 2 cm. The bar of tissue isolated between the two myotomies is resected with an angled rongeur introduced from the aorta, and usually also from the apical stab wound utilized for the left ventricular drain.

Thirty-seven of the 43 patients operated upon are living. Four hospital deaths resulted, respectively from arrhythmia, left ventricular failure, cerebral damage following an anaesthetic accident, and from the low output state in a boy in whom mitral valve replacement was required in addition to ventriculomyo-tomy. Two patients have died late of causes unrelated to their heart disease: one had a stroke, the other committed suicide. Two early patients (numbers 3 and 9 in the series) have complete heart block, and are maintained with implanted pacemakers. In one of these two patients a small interventricular septal defect was also created at operation; no attempt was made to close it, and the

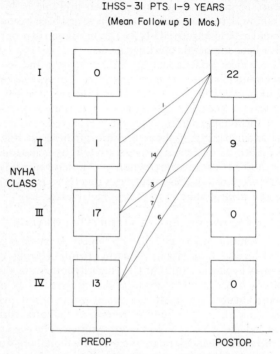

FIG. I. Functional classifications (New York Heart Association) of 31 patients with IHSS before and after operation. All patients have been followed more than one year, and the mean duration of follow-up is 51 months. The number within each box indicates the number of patients in that class.

resulting left-to-right shunt is small and requires no treatment. Two other patients in whom the operative procedure was uneventful were found to have interventricular septal defects at elective postoperative study. In each, an acute episode of failure and precordial pain suggested that the septum opened about six weeks postoperatively. Both patients are among the oldest operated upon, and it seems possible that in them the myotomy

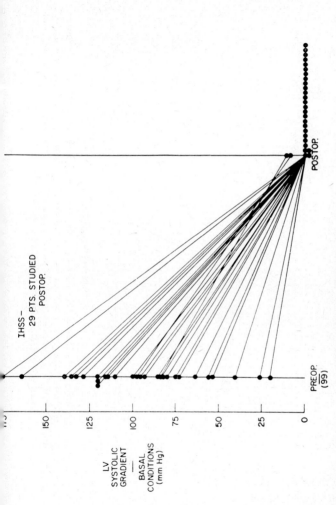

Fig. 1. Peak systolic pressure gradients between the left ventricle and the aorta or a peripheral artery recorded under basal conditions in 29 patients with IHSS studied before and after operation. No gradient was evident postoperatively in 27 patients, and in the other two the gradients were 11 and 8 mm Hg.

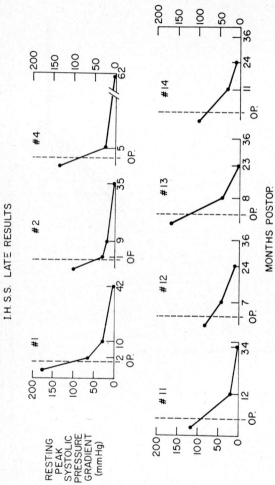

Fig. 3. Sequential measurements of the peak systolic pressure gradient between the left ventricle and a peripheral artery measured preoperatively (left of vertical dotted line) and at the postoperative intervals (months postop) indicated by the numerals. Observations were made in the seven patients who had residual obstruction at the initial postoperative study. See text for further explanation.

may have compromised an already diseased portion of the coronary circulation, with resulting septal infarction. Fortunately, in these two patients also the defects do not cause symptoms or significant haemodynamic abnormalities.

Thirty-one of the 37 surviving patients have been followed for at least one year, and for periods up to ten years; the mean duration of follow-up in the group is 51 months. The functional classifications of these 31 patients preoperatively and at most recent examination are shown graphically in Fig. 1.

### POSTOPERATIVE HAEMODYNAMIC EVALUATIONS

Left heart catheterization has been carried out on one or more occasions after operation in 29 patients. The peak systolic pressure gradients recorded at rest preoperatively and at latest postoperative study are plotted in Fig. 2.

The sequential haemodynamic findings in the seven patients who had evidence of some residual obstruction in the early postoperative period have been of particular interest. The preoperative and postoperative peak left ventriculo-aortic pressure gradients in these seven patients are plotted in Fig. 3. In five of the seven patients resting gradients were found five to 12 months after operation, but no gradients were evident at later studies. In the remaining two patients gradients of 44 and 30 mm Hg were present at seven and 11 months after operation, but had fallen to 11 and 8 mm Hg, respectively, at 24 months. It is noteworthy that in no patient has there been evidence of any recurrence or exacerbation of outflow obstruction at any time after operation.

In most patients, attempts have been made to determine not only the presence and magnitude of the pressure gradient at rest, but also during the application of provocative interventions. The gradients measured at rest and also during execution of the Valsalva manoeuvre or during isoprenaline (isoproterenol) infusion are plotted in Fig. 4. In 24 patients without resting gradients, gradients appeared with the Valsalva manoeuvre in 12, but only three exceeded 30 mm Hg. Isoprenaline was administered to 15 patients without resting gradients, and in nine of them gradients were provoked; only two exceeded 30 mm Hg, however. In the two patients with small resting gradients, the magnitude increased in both with the provocative test.

The left ventricular end-diastolic pressures recorded pre- and

IHSS—POSTOP PROVOCATIVE TESTS

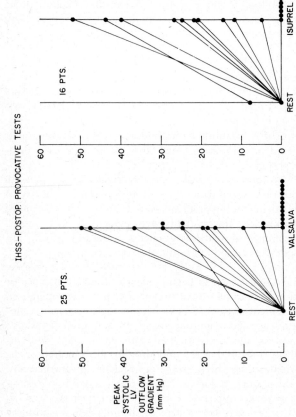

Fig. 4. Peak systolic pressure gradients between the left ventricle and a peripheral artery measured postoperatively in 25 patients before and during the Valsalva manoeuvre (left), and in 16 patients before and during isoprenaline (isoproterenol; Isuprel) administration (right).

postoperatively in 29 patients are plotted in Fig. 5. Preoperatively, the pressure was abnormally elevated (> 12 mm Hg) in 21 of the 29 patients. Postoperatively, the pressure decreased in 19 of the 21 in whom it had been abnormally high. In the entire group the mean value preoperatively was 20 mm Hg, and 12 mm Hg postoperatively.

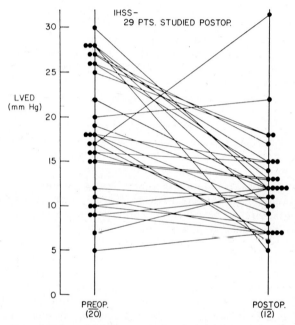

FIG. 5. Values of left ventricular end-diastolic pressure (LVED) recorded pre- and postoperatively in 29 patients with IHSS. Mean values are shown in parentheses.

The association of IHSS and mitral regurgitation is well recognized, and mitral regurgitation was evident preoperatively in 32 of the 37 patients in whom angiocardiograms or cineangiocardiograms of diagnostic quality were obtained. In 14 patients adequate left ventricular contrast studies were obtained both pre- and postoperatively, and mitral regurgitation was evident before operation in 13 of the 14. Postoperatively, the valve was seen to be completely competent in 11 of the 13, while in two patients mild mitral regurgitation persisted.

## COMMENT

When operation is contemplated in a patient with IHSS, and also when the results of operative treatment are evaluated, it must be borne in mind that there is no evidence that operation corrects the basic disease process, asymmetrical hypertrophy of the left ventricle. Thus, in patients without obstruction to left ventricular ejection, symptoms may result from decreased ventricular compliance, increased ventricular mass or impaired contractile function. The experience with these and other patients, however, indicates that operation can effectively relieve outflow obstruction, and thus relieve those symptoms caused by obstruction. In this clinic, operation was originally reserved for those patients with IHSS who were not only severely symptomatic but who also had severe obstruction when studied under resting basal conditions. With an improved understanding of the factors which regulate the contractile state of the myocardium, and consequently the severity of obstruction in IHSS, it has become apparent that in a significant number of patients no gradient is present at rest, but a large gradient may be induced by a number of interventions which reduce ventricular systolic volume. Also, it seems likely that in such patients severe symptoms may occur when obstruction is provoked by daily activities involving muscular exercise, postural changes, emotional stress, etc. For these reasons, operation has now been carried out in 11 patients in whom no gradient or a gradient less than 30 mm Hg was present before provocative interventions. Thus far the symptomatic improvement in these patients has paralleled that experienced by those with severe obstruction at rest, and this extension of the original indications for operation appears desirable.

## SUMMARY

The results of operative treatment (left ventriculomyotomy and myectomy) in 43 patients with idiopathic hypertrophic subaortic stenosis (IHSS) are described. All patients were severely symptomatic, and severe obstruction to left ventricular outflow was present under basal conditions (32 patients) or after various provocative interventions. Four patients died at or shortly after operation, and two patients have died late of causes unrelated to their cardiac disease.

Thirty-one of the 37 surviving patients have been followed for at least one year, and the mean follow-up period is 51 months. Twenty-two patients are now in functional Class I (NYHA), and nine are only mildly symptomatic (Class II). In 29 patients no resting intraventricular pressure gradient was present at post-operative left heart catheterization, and in the other two gradients of 11 and 8 mm Hg were recorded. The left ventricular end-diastolic pressure was lower postoperatively in 19 of the 21 patients in whom it had been abnormally elevated. Mitral regurgitation was abolished by operation in 11 of the 13 patients in whom comparative angiographic studies were made.

## REFERENCES

MORROW, A. G. (1969) *Archs Surg., Chicago* **99,** 677.
MORROW, A. G., FOGARTY, T. J., HANNAH, H. III and BRAUNWALD, E. (1968) *Circulation* **37,** 589.
MORROW, A. G., LAMBREW, C. T. and BRAUNWALD, E. (1964) In *Ciba Fdn Symp. Cardiomyopathies*, pp. 250–265. London: Churchill.

# SURGICAL TREATMENT OF IDIOPATHIC HYPER-TROPHIC SUBAORTIC STENOSIS USING A COMBINED LEFT VENTRICULAR-AORTIC APPROACH

B. G. BARRATT-BOYES
AND K. P. O'BRIEN

*Green Lane Hospital, Auckland*

OUR SURGICAL experience with idiopathic hypertrophic sub-aortic stenosis (IHSS) began in November 1960 using the myotomy incision advocated by Morrow and Braunwald (1959) and Cleland (1963). As Table I shows, the results in four patients were unsatisfactory, with one death after four months from unrelieved obstruction and three patients with important residual gradients which have subsequently been abolished by re-operation, using a combined left ventricular aortic approach. With myotomy, only two brothers (cases 5 and 6) have had a good result and in this familial pair the anterior muscular ridge was unusually discrete.

TABLE I

IHSS—MYOTOMY RESULTS

| Age (yr) and sex | Peak systolic gradient (mm Hg) | | Result |
|---|---|---|---|
| | Preoperative | Postoperative | |
| 54 M | 126 | 75 | |
| 32 M | 92 | 79 | Poor, re-operated |
| 35 F | 96 | 68 | |
| 40 F | 54 | — | |
| 10 M | 134 | 11 | Good |
| 14 M | 76 | 16 | |

Because of these unsatisfactory results with myotomy through an aortic approach, in December 1962 we began using the combined approach via the left ventricle and aorta (Kelly, Barratt-Boyes and Lowe 1966) described by Kirklin and Ellis (1961). In this presentation we report the results and follow-up in all 30 patients operated upon using this technique. Seventeen of these patients have been followed for from three to seven years.

## CLINICAL MATERIAL

The series consists of 12 males and 18 females aged 5 to 72 years. Five gave a familial history. The diagnosis of IHSS was made on clinical and haemodynamic criteria similar to those described by Braunwald and co-workers (1964). Operation was recommended in these patients chiefly because of an important left ventricular outflow gradient, particularly when this was combined with severe left ventricular hypertrophy on the electrocardiogram. Disabling symptoms were not a prerequisite, although they were usually present. Where case numbers are mentioned in the text they refer to the chronological order of operation on these patients.

## OPERATIVE TECHNIQUE

Under total body perfusion the nasopharyngeal temperature was lowered to 28 °C to allow aortic cross-clamping without coronary perfusion for 20 to 30 minutes and to provide a completely relaxed myocardium, which is considered essential if a ventriculotomy is used. The aorta was opened through a vertical incision, passing downwards into the non-coronary sinus of Valsalva, and excision of the anterior muscular bar commenced from above. At this stage, before dislocating the heart forwards for the left ventricular incision and to avoid air embolization to the right coronary artery during this manoeuvre, both coronary arteries were cannulated. Once the cannulae were in position, perfusion through them was stopped to ensure a completely relaxed fibrillating heart during the next phase.

The left ventricle was then opened through an oblique incision on the lower antero-lateral wall, entering the ventricle medial to the anterior papillary muscle. Muscle was excised from the anterior portion of the septum, creating a deep wide trough which became continuous with the anterior wedge already removed from above.

Coronary artery perfusion was commenced as the patient was rewarmed and the ventricular and aortic incisions were closed, using interrupted full thickness sutures for the former.

## MORTALITY

In this group of 30 operated patients there was one hospital death from dehiscence of the ventriculotomy, due probably to insecure initial closure.

6

In addition, there were two late deaths. A 14-year-old boy died suddenly four months postoperatively while running up the school stairs, presumably from arrhythmia. His postoperative electrocardiogram was consistent with antero-lateral myocardial infarction, although at autopsy scarring was confined to the

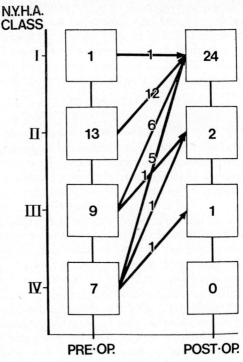

Fig. 1. Symptomatic limitation in 30 patients.

immediate vicinity of the ventricular incision and the obstruction was adequately relieved. The second late death occurred 13 months postoperatively from a sudden severe hemiparesis in a 37-year-old woman who was in chronic atrial fibrillation pre- and postoperatively. At autopsy an embolus was found occluding the right internal carotid artery. No intracardiac thrombus was demonstrated and the obstruction had been adequately relieved.

## MORBIDITY

Two patients operated upon early in the series (cases 3 and 4) have developed a left ventricular aneurysm at the ventriculotomy site. In case 3 the aneurysm was repaired uneventfully 17 months postoperatively and this patient is asymptomatic. In case 4 the aneurysm has gradually calcified and although it is associated with a raised left ventricular end-diastolic pressure of 20 mm Hg and interstitial oedema on the chest radiograph, the patient is completely symptom-free seven years postoperatively and has not therefore been re-operated upon.

There has been no other important morbidity; in particular, no patient has surgically induced complete heart block, ventricular septal defect or aortic incompetence.

It is worthy of comment that in the first half of this series, when the importance of avoiding coronary air embolization during the ventriculotomy was not appreciated, a low output state with hypotension and ventricular irritability was not uncommon in the early postoperative period. This situation has not been encountered since correcting this error in technique.

## COMPARISON OF PRE- AND POSTOPERATIVE STATUS

*Symptoms* (Fig. 1)

After operation all symptomatic patients have shown improvement and in most this benefit has been striking. Twenty-four of the 27 long-term survivors are completely symptom-free; two are now Class II (New York Heart Association) (one with mild angina and one with mild effort dyspnoea), but neither has a significant outflow gradient (0 and 14 mm Hg) and one is now Class III, but this man (case 30) was in congestive heart failure and atrial fibrillation, and was operated upon only eight months ago. Postoperatively he remains in atrial fibrillation and, although the outflow gradient has been abolished, he has residual moderate mitral incompetence.

*Electrocardiogram*

Before operation four patients had complete left bundle branch block. After operation 11 patients developed complete

left bundle branch block as a new feature and a further 11 developed
left axis deviation with a widened QRS (less than 0·12 s duration).
Two patients in atrial fibrillation preoperatively remained in this
rhythm, while all others have remained in sinus rhythm. Neither
patient with persistent atrial fibrillation has done well; one died

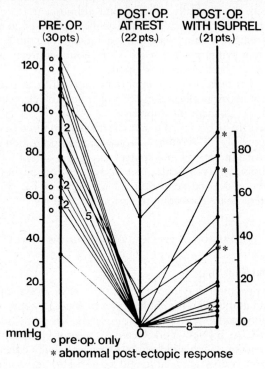

FIG. 2. Left ventricular outflow gradients before and after
operation.

from a cerebral embolus and the other (case 30) has persistent
symptoms.

Postoperatively three patients developed changes consistent
with myocardial infarction (antero-lateral in two and posterior
in one). One of these died suddenly four months postoperatively
from arrhythmia; the other two are symptom-free.

## Haemodynamic studies

Before operation cardiac catheterization was performed in each patient. The resting left ventricular outflow peak systolic pressure gradients ranged from 34 to 125 mm Hg and averaged 85 mm Hg. Four patients had additional right ventricular outflow gradients ranging from 24 to 34 mm Hg.

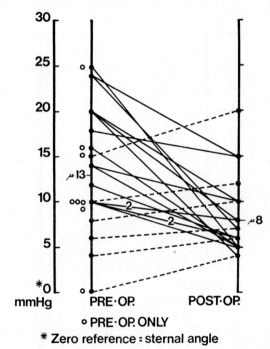

FIG. 3. Left ventricular end-diastolic pressures before and after operation in 22 patients.

Twenty-two of the 27 survivors had one postoperative catheter and in six of these a second study was performed two to four years after the first. In the six with two studies the gradient at the second study has remained the same or decreased in five, and increased slightly in one.

After operation the resting gradient was abolished in 18 of the 22 patients (Fig. 2). In two the gradient was less than 20 mm Hg;

in one studied one year postoperatively it measured 50 mm Hg and in one, studied at five years, 60 mm Hg.

In 21 of the 22 an attempt was made to provoke an outflow gradient (using Isuprel [isoprenaline] in 19, exercise in one and the Valsalva manoeuvre in one). This resulted in a gradient greater than 20 mm Hg in six.

The post-ectopic response returned to normal in all patients studied except three (Fig. 2). The left ventricular end-diastolic

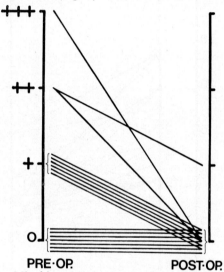

**PRE·OP.**                              **POST·OP.**

FIG. 4. Mitral regurgitation in 16 patients before and after operation.

pressure averaged 13 mm Hg preoperatively, and postoperatively, when this pressure remained above 10 mm Hg in only four, it averaged 8 mm Hg (Fig. 3). None of these four patients has an outflow gradient above 10 mm Hg either at rest or on Isuprel administration and none has residual mitral incompetence on angiocardiography. Only one patient shows a significant rise in pressure postoperatively (to 20 mm Hg) and this is associated with a residual left ventricular aneurysm (case 4).

*Left ventricular angiography*

Eighteen of 21 patients who had a postoperative angiocardiographic study have no mitral incompetence, two have mild incompetence and one moderate incompetence. The single patient with residual moderate incompetence (case 30) did not have an angiocardiogram preoperatively and has been studied for only eight months postoperatively. He has no residual gradient and a normal left ventricular end-diastolic pressure but

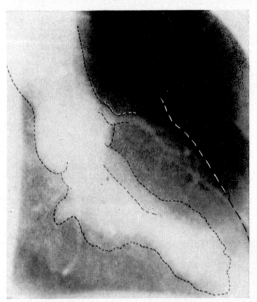

Fig. 5. Shallow right anterior oblique left ventricular cine frame in systole, showing the surgical groove which appears as a double contour of the leftward anterior margin of the outflow tract.

remains symptomatic. The changes recorded in the 16 with both pre- and postoperative angiograms are shown in Fig. 4.

In the postoperative angiocardiogram, the surgical groove cut in the antero-lateral wall of the left ventricular outflow tract connecting the body of the ventricle to the subaortic region was visible in 18 of the 21 patients (Fig. 5). At the ventriculotomy site there was a muscle recess in 11 patients (Fig. 6). This recess was distinguishable from an aneurysm on the cine studies by both a reduction in size and some increase in thickness of the muscle overlying it during systole.

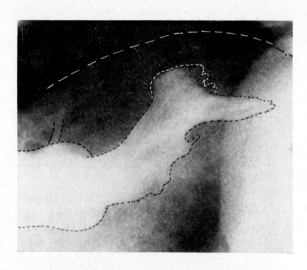
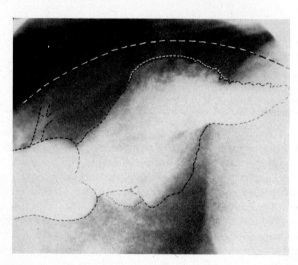

FIG. 6. Shallow right anterior oblique left ventricular cine frame showing a recess at the ventriculotomy site which becomes smaller during systole. Left—diastole; right—systole.

## SUMMARY AND CONCLUSIONS

The follow-up of 30 patients with idiopathic hypertrophic subaortic stenosis (IHSS) operated upon using a combined left ventricular aortic approach is presented. Seventeen of the 27 survivors have been followed for three to seven years. There has been only one hospital death from surgical error, namely rupture of the left ventricular incision. There have been two late deaths, one from cerebral embolus unrelated to the procedure and one from arrhythmia, doubtfully related although the postoperative electrocardiogram showed changes consistent with antero-lateral infarction.

All 27 survivors have shown symptomatic improvement, usually striking, and only three have residual symptoms. Only two patients of the 22 recatheterized have significant residual resting outflow gradients and both are asymptomatic. Morbidity has been confined to two early patients who developed a left ventricular aneurysm.

It is concluded that this procedure can be relied upon to abolish or significantly reduce the obstructive element in this disease and will also usually lower the left ventricular end-diastolic pressure and abolish mitral incompetence. For these reasons it is considered to be clearly indicated in patients with obstruction and disabling symptoms and is probably indicated in all patients with an important outflow gradient. In our hands the combined left ventricular-aortic approach has been associated with a low mortality and morbidity and has given results superior to those using an aortic approach alone.

## REFERENCES

BRAUNWALD, E., LAMBREW, C. T., ROCKOFF, S. D., ROSS, J. JR and MORROW, A. G. (1964) *Circulation* 30, Suppl. IV, 3–213.

CLELAND, W. P. (1963) *J. cardiovasc. Surg.* 4, 489–494.

KELLY, D. T., BARRATT-BOYES, B. G. and LOWE, J. B. (1966) *J. thorac. cardiovasc. Surg.* 51, 353–365.

KIRKLIN, J. W. and ELLIS, F. H. JR. (1961) *Circulation* 24, 739–742.

MORROW, A. G. and BRAUNWALD, E. (1959) *Circulation* 20, 181–189.

# TREATMENT OF HYPERTROPHIC OBSTRUCTIVE CARDIOMYOPATHY BY SEPTECTOMY

E. van de Wall
AND J. N. Homan van der Heide

*Department of Cardiology and Department of Thoracic Surgery,
University Hospital, Groningen*

THE surgical relief of left ventricular outflow obstruction in hypertrophic obstructive cardiomyopathy (HOCM) is based on a combination of two surgical possibilities: myotomy and myectomy.

Myotomy with limited myectomy as described by Braunwald and co-workers (1964), Morrow, Lambrew and Braunwald (1964), Morrow and co-workers (1968), Cleland (1963, 1964), Cleland and co-workers (1969), Bentall (1964) and Bentall and co-workers (1965), has given discouraging results in our hands. We found it difficult to estimate the depth of the myotomy and the amount of muscle to be resected. Bidigital exploration of the hypertrophic septum through a combined aortic and right ventricular approach as described by Cooley and co-workers (1967) permitted us to localize the obstruction more exactly and resect it completely.

### OPERATIVE TECHNIQUE

Fig. 1 shows the operation schematically. After institution of normothermic cardiopulmonary bypass, the ascending aorta is cross-clamped and opened by a small transverse incision. The left index finger is then inserted into the left ventricle. A small transverse incision is made in the right ventricle and the hyper-trophied septum is pushed upwards. The hypertrophy is now clearly seen and can be resected with a cutting spoon-like forceps, as shown in Fig. 1. Guided by bidigital palpation, a myectomy can be performed which encompasses the full width and length of the obstruction. The thickness of the septum is reduced until 0·5 cm is still present between the two palpating fingers.

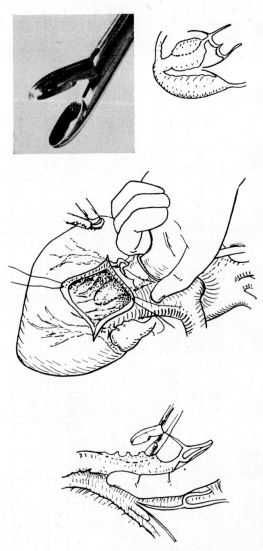

FIG. 1. Operation technique.

TABLE I

SYMPTOMS, CLINICAL SIGNS, LEFT VENTRICULO-AORTIC GRADIENT AT REST AND FUNCTIONAL CLASSIFICATION (N.Y.H.A.)
FOR EVERY PATIENT BEFORE (LEFT COLUMN) AND AFTER OPERATION (RIGHT COLUMN)

| | 1 J.A-V. 41F | 2 A.B. 34M | 3 W.deB. 47M | 4 G.D. 34F | 5 H.H-K 40F | 6 B.R. 39M | 7 G.R. 48M | 8 T.K-V. 51F |
|---|---|---|---|---|---|---|---|---|
| **A) SYMPTOMS** | | | | | | | | |
| dyspnoea | | | | | | | | |
| angina pectoris | | | | | | | | |
| dizziness | | | | | | | | |
| syncope | | | | | | | | |
| palpitations | | | | | | | | |
| fatigue | | | | | | | | |
| oedema | | | | | | | | |
| **B) SIGNS** | | | | | | | | |
| SEM, L.S.E. | | | | | | | | |
| thrill | | | | | | | | |
| double apex beat | | | | | | | | |
| R.V. impulse | | | | | | | | |
| M.I. | | | | | | | | |
| IV sound | | | | | | | | |
| L.V.H. | | | | | | | | |
| rhythm | sinus / sinus | sinus / sinus | Atr. Fibr. / sinus | sinus / sinus | sinus / sinus | sinus / sinus | sinus | sinus |
| **C) L.V.-Ao. pressure gradient at rest** | 100 | 70 | 75 / 0 | 115 | 110 | 40 | 100 | 50 |
| **D) Functional classification (N.Y.H.A.)** | III / I | III / I | III / I | III / II | III / II | III / I | IV | IV |

□ = No symptoms or signs present; ■ = presence of symptoms and signs at rest and on exertion; ▨ = presence of symptoms and

## RESULTS

Eight patients were operated on in this way. The weight of the resected tissue varied in these cases from 3 g to 12 g. The period of aortic occlusion and myocardial ischaemia ranged from 12 to 33 minutes. In none of the patients did heart block occur.

The indications for operation depend on progression of long-standing symptoms in spite of intensive medication with propranolol (Inderal), familial occurrence, and a gradient exceeding 50 mm Hg at rest. Table I shows the signs and symptoms in our eight patients before and after operation. Two patients (nos. 7 and 8) died immediately after the operation from a low output syndrome. The remaining six cases are still alive from 13 to 28 months after operation.

Our follow-up disclosed that all patients showed subjective improvement. In four the improvement was such as to permit them to resume normal work. Two patients (nos. 4 and 5) improved after the operations but in view of their symptoms they still had to be classified in Class II (N.Y.H.A.).

The question arises of whether adequate removal of obstruction was obtained. Because recatheterization should not be done until eight to 12 months after operation and the most suitable patients refused this type of re-evaluation, only one patient (no. 3) in whom good clinical results were obtained could be evaluated in this way. The withdrawal tracings in Fig. 2 show that the pressure gradient completely disappeared after operation in this patient and the cardiac index increased from 2·30 l/min per square metre to 3·27 l/min per square metre. The angiocardiogram, taken in the right anterior oblique position (Fig. 3), shows clearly that the obstruction was removed by myectomy. However a small ventricular septal defect with a haemodynamically unimportant shunt (20 per cent) occurred in this patient.

Removal of the obstruction can also be evaluated by other less traumatic parameters, such as external carotid tracings, apex cardiograms and phonocardiograms. Table II shows that the ejection times, measured from external carotid curves and corrected for heart rate according to Weissler (1963), differ from the normal values of 396 ms (±0·0145) for males and 411 ms (± 0·1016) for females (Weissler 1963). However, all our patients had received the β-blocking agent propranolol (Inderal), which prolongs the ejection time intervals, for some considerable time

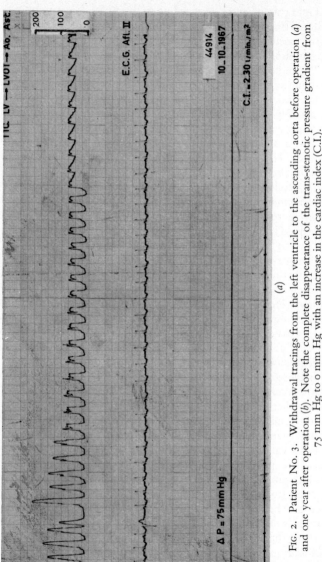

FIG. 2. Patient No. 3. Withdrawal tracings from the left ventricle to the ascending aorta before operation (*a*) and one year after operation (*b*). Note the complete disappearance of the trans-stenotic pressure gradient from 75 mm Hg to o mm Hg with an increase in the cardiac index (C.I.).

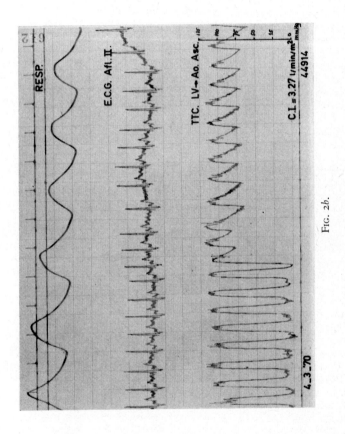

FIG. 2b.

## TABLE II

EJECTION TIME INTERVALS, TRANS-STENOTIC PRESSURE GRADIENTS, A-WAVE RATIO (A/H) AND LEFT VENTRICULAR END-DIASTOLIC PRESSURE (LVEDP)

| Pat. | Age/sex | F/S | Ejection time (ms) corrected for heart rate | | LV-Ao gradient at rest (mm Hg) | | A/H ratio (%) | | LVEDP (mm Hg) | |
|---|---|---|---|---|---|---|---|---|---|---|
| 1. J.A.-V. | 41 F | F | 434 | 464 | 110 | — | 28 | 15 | 30 | — |
| 2. A.B. | 34 M | F | 432 | 412 | 70 | — | 40 | 18 | 35 | — |
| 3. W.B. | 47 M | F | 436 | 322 | 75 | 0 | 27 | — | 30 | 10 |
| 4. G.D. | 34 F | F | 426 | 444 | 115 | — | 21 | 23 | 25 | — |
| 5. H.H.-K. | 38 F | S | 456 | 413 | 110 | — | 17 | 16 | 25 | — |
| 6. B.R. | 39 M | F | 440 | 408 | 40 | — | 26 | 18 | 25 | — |

Left column before, right column after operation.
Patients 3 and 6 did not receive propranolol postoperatively.
F/S: familial or sporadic case.

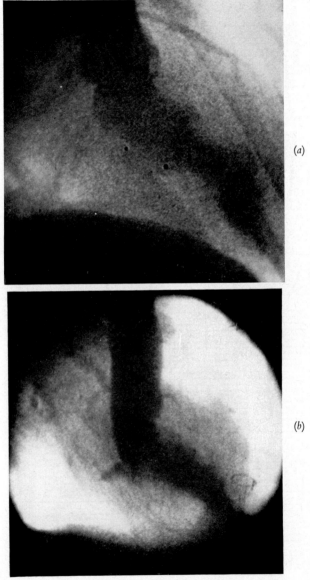

(a)

(b)

FIG. 3. Patient No. 3. Angiocardiogram of the left ventricle in systole taken in the right anterior oblique position before (a) and one year after operation (b). (Recorded at the Radiological Institute, University Hospital, Groningen.)

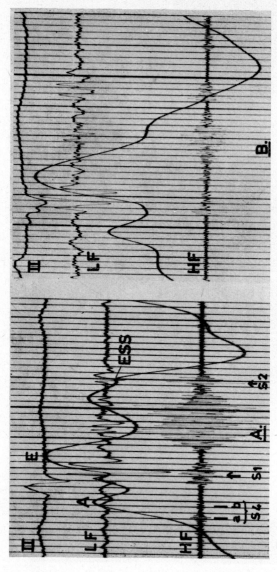

FIG. 4.  Patient No. 2.  Apex cardiogram (ACG) before (A) and after operation (B).  The two components of the fourth heart sound (S4 a, b) in the high frequency band (HF = 140 Hz) have disappeared after operation with a reduction of the A-wave ratio from 40% to 18%.  II: ECG lead II; A: A-wave of the ACG; E: ejection point of the ACG; ESS: end-systolic shoulder of the ACG.

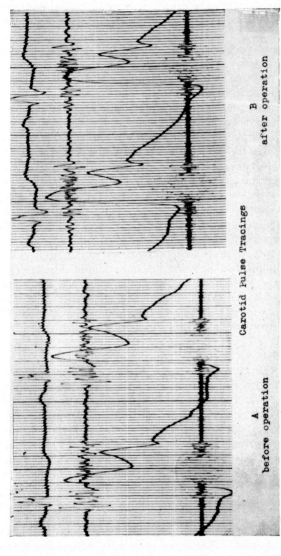

FIG. 5. Patient No. 6. External carotid pulse tracings before (A) and 20 months after (B) operation. The well-developed tidal wave is still present after operation, the corresponding ejection time indices being 440 ms and 408 ms respectively.

before the operation, so that what would otherwise have been a direct relation between the degree of obstruction and the prolongation of the ejection time (Wigle *et al.* 1968) had been disturbed.

Four patients (nos. 1, 2, 4, 5) were given propranolol postoperatively, chiefly to suppress slight attacks of palpitations. Though in two (nos. 1 and 2) the clinical result was excellent, no significant reduction of the left ventricular ejection time occurred. Patients nos. 3 and 6, who required no postoperative propranolol medication, showed a decrease in ejection time; this applies in particular to patient no. 3, in whom recatheterization showed that the pressure gradient had disappeared.

Table II also shows that the patients who were asymptomatic after the operation (nos. 1, 2, 6) showed a significant reduction in percentage of the A-wave ratio of the apical pulse tracing. The apex cardiogram of patient no. 2 (Fig. 4) is a typical example of the postoperative changes to be obtained with this operation. Unfortunately, the only patient who was catheterized postoperatively (no. 3) developed postoperative atrial fibrillation. Electrical defibrillation failed to restore sinus rhythm. The A-wave ratio therefore could not be assessed, but there was a marked decrease in left ventricular end-diastolic pressure. The two patients whose postoperative N.Y.H.A. classification was Class II (nos. 4 and 5) showed no change in percentage of the A-wave ratio.

As demonstrated by other investigators (Epstein *et al.* 1968; Nagle *et al.* 1966), the height of the A-wave of the apex cardiogram reflects increased atrial transport as a result of diminished compliance of the left ventricle. In our series the presence of a large A-wave invariably coincided with a marked fourth sound, the latter being present in both the lower (35, 70 Hz) and the higher (140, 250 Hz) frequency bands. With a postoperative decrease in percentage of the A-wave ratio the amplitude of the fourth sound in the lower frequencies was concomitantly reduced and it disappeared completely in the higher frequencies.

These findings may lend some support to the conclusion that in our series, in the three patients in whom the A-wave ratio was markedly reduced, the atrial drive had been reduced by the mechanical removal of obstruction of the left ventricular outflow tract.

In our experience and that of many other investigators, neither the external carotid pulse tracing nor the changes in the systolic ejection murmur gave any reliable information about the benefit derived from the operation. In most cases the bifid carotid arterial tracing persisted after the operation (Fig. 5), and the systolic ejection murmur and signs of left ventricular hypertrophy were still present after the operation, although the systolic murmur was of somewhat lower intensity and shorter duration.

## CONCLUSIONS

In summarizing the results we may state that:

(a) In one patient (no. 3) removal of the obstruction was obtained with certainty according to recatheterization data;

(b) In three patients (nos. 1, 2, 6), according to the clinical results, the concomitant reduction of the A-wave ratios and the left ventricular ejection times, adequate removal of obstruction is highly probable but must be verified by recatheterization;

(c) In two patients (nos. 4 and 5) surgical removal of obstruction may have failed. But we must remember that relief of the outflow block does not imply relief of the inflow block, even though the mechanical removal of obstruction may have a favourable effect on the remaining cardiopathy.

However, our series of patients is too small to warrant comparison with the much larger series of Braunwald and co-workers (1964) and Goodwin and others (Bentall et al. 1965). Although very encouraging results were obtained in four of our eight patients, two (nos. 7 and 8) died from the intervention. These were the oldest patients in our series (48 and 51 years, respectively) and both had had serious symptoms for years, probably caused not only by a local obstruction but also by an advanced cardiomyopathy. The operation performed, which effected only mechanical removal of obstruction, undoubtedly came too late in these two cases. We cannot escape the impression that in these cases the removal of obstruction merely unmasked the concomitant cardiomyopathy.

In conclusion we may state that myectomy guided by bidigital palpation can effect adequate removal of obstruction. Whether this procedure yields better results than transaortic myotomy with limited myectomy cannot yet be established with certainty.

SUMMARY

Myotomy with limited myectomy as described by other workers has given us discouraging results in the surgical relief of left ventricular outflow obstruction caused by hypertrophic obstructive cardiomyopathy. It was difficult to estimate the depth of the myotomy and the amount of muscle to be resected. Bidigital exploration of the hypertrophic septum through a combined aortic and right ventricular approach, as described by Cooley and co-workers (1967), permits of exact localization and careful resection of the entire obstruction.

Eight patients were treated by this procedure; two died in the immediate postoperative period from a low output syndrome. Both belonged to the older group and their severe myopathy may have caused the fatal issue.

Of the six surviving patients, four improved considerably and were able to resume work. The objective and subjective signs of improvement are discussed. Our series is still too small for these extended myectomies through the right ventricle to be compared with other surgical procedures. However, the Cooley-type operation may give very satisfactory results, although in severe myopathy a myectomy may well be contraindicated.

REFERENCES

BENTALL, H. H. (1964) In *Ciba Fdn Symp. Cardiomyopathies*, pp. 272–275. London: Churchill.

BENTALL, H. H., CLELAND, W. P., OAKLEY, C. M., SHAH, P. M., STEINER, R. E. and GOODWIN, J. F. (1965) *Br. Heart J.* **27**, 585–594.

BRAUNWALD, E., LAMBREW, C. T., ROCKOFF, S. O., ROSS, J. and MORROW, A. G. (1964) *Circulation* **30**, Suppl. IV, 3–119.

CLELAND, W. P. (1963) *J. cardiovasc. Surg.* **4**, 489–491.

CLELAND, W. P. (1964) In *Ciba Fdn Symp. Cardiomyopathies*, pp. 276–284. London: Churchill.

CLELAND, W. P., GOODWIN, J. F., MCDONALD, L. and ROSS, D. (1969) In *Medical and Surgical Cardiology*, pp. 951–978. Oxford and Edinburgh: Blackwell Scientific Publications.

COOLEY, D. H., BLOODWELL, R. D., HALLMAN, G. L., LA SORTE, A., LEACHMAN, R. D. and CHAPMAN, D. W. (1967) *Circulation* **35**, Suppl. I, 124–132.

EPSTEIN, E. J., COULSHED, N., BROWN, A. K. and DOUKAS, N. G. (1968) *Br. Heart J.* **30**, 591–605.

MORROW, A. G., FOGARTY, T. J., HANNAH, I. H. and BRAUNWALD, E. (1968) *Circulation* **37**, 589–596.

MORROW, A. G., LAMBREW, C. T. and BRAUNWALD, E. (1964) In *Ciba Fdn Symp. Cardiomyopathies*, pp. 250–265. London: Churchill.
NAGLE, R. E., BOICOURT, O. W., GILLAM, P. M. S. and MOUNSEY, J. P. D. (1966) *Br. Heart J.* **28**, 419–425.
WEISSLER, A. M. (1963) *J. appl. Physiol.* **18**, 919–922.
WIGLE, E. D., TRIMBLE, A. S., ADELMAN, A. G. and BIGELOW, W. G. (1968) *Prog. cardiovasc. Dis.* **11**, 2, 83–112.

## DISCUSSION

*Cleland:* This follow-up to the Ciba Foundation symposium in 1964 gives us an opportunity of comparing our thoughts in 1964 with those of 1970. With regard to surgical management we should ask four succinct questions: 'If', 'When', 'How', and 'With what results?'. In 1964 the main requirement for surgery was the presence of a gradient either at rest or provoked by isoprenaline. Less importance was placed on the presence of symptoms. Today we must have a gradient of some severity but are much more concerned about the presence of symptoms, because we have found that surgery is really a very effective way of relieving them. From our own experience we cannot be certain yet that life is prolonged but all our results indicate that surgery has given excellent relief of the symptoms. This, of course, must partly or wholly be associated with the elimination of the obstruction, and with it the gradient. However, one very important by-product of surgery, and probably very relevant to the relief of symptoms, has been the reduction or elimination of mitral regurgitation. Everyone has had this experience, whatever method has been used to relieve the obstruction. Whatever the mechanism of production of mitral regurgitation it seems that the final mechanism must be the difference in the pressures on the two sides of the aortic leaflet of the mitral valve during ventricular systole. This differential should disappear after successful surgery.

With regard to 'How', most of the early surgical procedures should be described as a ventricular myotomy. Certainly the first 10 or 12 patients that Bentall and I operated on had what could only be described as a ventricular myotomy, and a very limited one at that. In 1964 this was still our view, but we had a general feeling of unhappiness about ventricular myotomy alone. Our own experience at Hammersmith had not been entirely happy; a number of patients were left with gradients of some severity, and relief of symptoms was variable. Since 1964 we have been using a combined aortic and ventricular approach as advocated by Kirklin and used and described here by Barratt-Boyes. However, Glen Morrow has continued to employ an aortic approach with ventricular myotomy without essential modification. His results are probably the best in the world, and I think this is an important message. In this connexion I would like to remind you that the first patient ever to be deliberately operated on for this condition had a very limited ventricular myotomy in 1958 at Hammersmith and is still remarkably fit, well and symptom-free today. I personally am veering back to the original aortic approach with a simple ventricular myotomy. However, John Kirklin's approach is impressive and more satisfying for a surgeon to do, and on the few occasions I have used it I have felt very much happier about what I had been able to achieve. Our own experience with techniques other than ventriculomyotomy through the aorta has indicated that the complications and especially rhythm disturbances are higher. Barratt-Boyes has hinted that this may be due to air getting into the coronaries and perhaps his technique of preventing this with cannulation of the coronaries before the heart is up-ended is important.

*Barratt-Boyes:* I understand that in many patients Dr Morrow added a blind approach via the apex of the left ventricle to complete the excision of muscle.

*Braunwald:* I don't believe so.

*O'Brien:* I don't think I saw him use an approach from the apex but I could not be sure of this. I don't think, Dr Braunwald, that you need worry about dissociating yourself from those patients who had small gradients or no gradients, because these are excellent results (Epstein and Morrow 1970). About four that I remember had small gradients or no gradient at rest. One in particular had a resting gradient of 15 mm Hg and gross mitral regurgitation, and was grossly limited. All she had was the standard Morrow operation and afterwards symptomatically she was markedly improved and mitral regurgitation was abolished.

*Olsen:* Dr Braunwald, you did not mention left bundle branch block when you discussed the complications. Did this occur in many of these patients?

*Braunwald:* Left bundle block occurred in almost every patient. We didn't include that as a complication because we thought it had little clinical importance. The incision on the left ventricular aspect of the septum which causes the left bundle branch block is also responsible, we feel, for the relief of obstruction. The bundle branch block appears to be incidental.

*Nellen:* How did the heart block patients progress?

*Braunwald:* There were two such patients and they had pace-makers inserted.

*Burchell:* Left bundle branch block is not necessarily a conse-quence of an operation in the bulging septum, because one would ordinarily make the excision, as Dr Morrow does, anterior to the first branches of the left bundle system. We have more often seen an anterior fasciculus block, and perhaps only about 25 per cent with left bundle branch block.

*Wigle:* Of the 27 patients Dr Bigelow has operated on, three or four had no conduction defect whatsoever. About 21 out of 27 had the anterior division block producing left axis deviation and only two or three had left bundle branch block. These observa-tions suggest that it is not the conduction defects that cause the beneficial results of the surgery.

*Nellen:* Dr Barratt-Boyes, did you produce complete heart block in any of the patients that you operated on?

*Barratt-Boyes:* No.

*Shah:* As alluded to earlier (p. 101), we have had an opportunity to study 14 patients by ultrasound method after surgery. In striking contrast to the untreated group of patients, the systolic abnormality of mitral valve motion was absent at rest in 11 cases (see Table I, p. 125). Independent haemodynamic studies before and after surgery were done in nine of these 14 patients (Fig. 1). Seven of these had no ultrasound abnormality at rest, five having no resting gradients and two a peak outflow gradient of 10 mm Hg. Two patients with ultrasound abnormality at rest also had significant gradients at rest. Ability of appropriate interventions (e.g. Valsalva manoeuvre, post-ectopic response, amyl nitrite, isoproterenol [isoprenaline]) to provoke outflow gradients correlated with the development of ultrasound abnormality on provocation.

We have also examined the diastolic function of the left ventricle as reflected in the mitral valve motion. The slope of the posterior movement EF in early diastole reflects the rate of rapid ventricular filling. This slope is markedly reduced in patients with mitral stenosis. We have observed considerable reduction in this slope EF in the presence of gross left ventricular hypertrophy and have

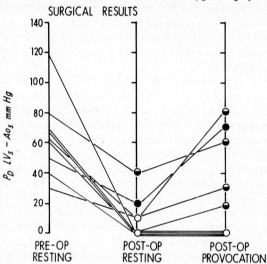

FIG. 1 (Shah). Correlation of pressure gradients obtained at the haemodynamic evaluation after surgery with the ultrasound findings in mitral valve motion both at rest and on provocation.

interpreted it to mean reduced ventricular distensibility with impaired diastolic filling (Shah et al. 1968). Analysis of the EF slope in patients with HOCM revealed that those with persistent and complete systolic abnormality had the most pronounced reduction in slope EF, many falling in the range that has been considered diagnostic for mitral stenosis. In contrast the patients with no abnormalities in the systolic segment of mitral valve motion generally had more rapid slopes, often in the normal range. Most of these patients had no evidence of resting obstruction on haemodynamic studies and had undergone successful surgical relief of outflow obstruction. Thus it is felt that the presence of persistent outflow obstruction is more generally associated with more severe impairment in diastolic filling of the left ventricle. The mechanisms by which the abnormal mitral valve motion may result in outflow obstruction in systole and by which this abnormality is correlated after surgical relief of obstruction are not clearly understood. However, these observations document the functional role of the mitral valve in outflow obstruction and mitral regurgitation, two important features of this entity.

*Silver:* In Toronto we have been interested in the pattern of distribution of the bizarre muscle in HOCM. Dr Shah in 1964 reported a patient with cardiomyopathy in whom the middle circular and superficial oblique muscle layers were markedly hypertrophied. To determine whether a particular muscle bundle, in the Mall tradition (Mall 1911), was affected in HOCM we studied the distribution of the bizarre muscle in the hearts of seven patients; six had had subaortic stenosis demonstrated clinically, while no obstruction could be demonstrated in the seventh. Six of the hearts were cross-sectioned into slices 1 cm thick proceeding from their apex to the base. Contiguous histological blocks were taken from the basal surface of each slice to include all of its surface area. The distribution of the bizarre muscle pattern was determined microscopically and mapped to scale on pieces of paper subsequently arranged to provide a three-dimensional impression of the distribution. The other heart was sliced longitudinally from anterior to posterior surface. Again histological blocks were prepared from the anterior surface of each slice and a paper map prepared.

The muscle in the ventricular wall can be divided into three artificial layers of epicardial, middle and endocardial fasciculi, depending upon the direction the fibres run (Lev and Simpkins 1956). The bizarre muscle in the seven hearts formed a band of circumferentially running fibres in the mid-third of the ventricular wall. The band was limited almost entirely to the left ventricular wall but had short projections into the mid-third of the right ventricular wall at its junctions with the septum. Furthermore, the band in the left ventricle widened as it proceeded from apex to base and from it bizarre fibres could be traced towards the endocardial surface, even extending into the papillary muscles and towards the epicardial surface. Other hearts hypertrophied as a result of valvular disease or hypertension were also examined in this manner. In them occasional focal areas of bizarre muscle fibres were found distributed in an irregular fashion in the left ventricular wall, usually towards the base of the heart; however, the pattern of distribution was never as constant as that seen in hearts with HOCM.

The findings indicate that a circumferentially running group of fibres in the mid-part of the left ventricular wall are the ones principally affected in HOCM. They agree with the concept Professor Bentall mentioned that the origin of the left ventricular muscle differs from that of the right. However, the distribution of the affected muscle does not correspond exactly with any of the muscle bundles Mall described.

*Braunwald:* In 1964 Dr Morrow reported the first ten of the 43 patients discussed here (Morrow, Lambrew and Braunwald 1964). In all ten the approach was through the aorta, in five there was a myotomy and in another five a limited myectomy. In most of the later 33 patients the incision was the same, through the aorta, but there was a limited myectomy in addition to a deep incision.

*Cleland:* One obvious difference is that the original myotomy was made with a single incision deepened by the finger, and the present technique consists of a double incision with the removal of the central core of muscle.

*Wigle:* Dr Bigelow has used only the ventriculomyotomy incision without removal of muscle in operating on 25 patients (and two later ones). Three of the 25 were in Class II preoperatively; postoperatively two went into Class I and one remained in Class II. Twenty patients were Class III–IV at the time of operation: five are Class I postoperatively, 11 are Class II and one remains unchanged. There were three operative deaths, giving an operative mortality of 12 per cent, or 11 per cent if the two additional cases are included. There were three late deaths: one man died from aspiration during gall bladder surgery in a small hospital five years after surgery, after being completely asymptomatic; one fell off a roof four years after the operation, possibly as the result of arrhythmia, and one poisoned himself with digitalis. Nearly all the cases that were in Class I postoperatively were recatheterized and in most we could not stimulate gradients. End-diastolic pressure was reduced in all except one. In those in Class II or III postoperatively the gradient was again usually abolished at rest, but in these it could often be stimulated; the end-diastolic pressures basically went down except in two cases who were not improved by the surgery. Simple myotomy, then, is effective. Dr Morrow started with myotomy and yet went on to use a slight myectomy as well, and other surgeons have gone on to various other forms of resection, but in fact seemingly adequate operative results can be obtained when the muscle is simply incised to a sufficient depth in the correct place.

*Braunwald:* I think that Mr Cleland and Mr Bentall started the myotomy because it was after his return from Hammersmith Hospital that Glen Morrow did his first operation and indicated that he was following their lead.

*Oakley:* In a progressive disease we must have good evidence either that the function of the disordered left ventricle is being improved by the operation or that the expected future deterioration is going to be prevented or delayed. All patients improve after cardiac operations, and if they have a rare disease they improve even more. We know that the left ventricular outflow tract obstruction tends to disappear anyway, and maybe operation actually hastens the downward progress of the disease by incurring further muscle damage rather than improving function. I will let a skeleton out of our cupboard by admitting that in one of the patients who lost outflow tract obstruction (and lost the systolic opening movement on the ultrasound records) this 'improvement' was achieved by infarcting the ventricle. This occurred through dissection of the anterior descending branch of the left coronary artery. This patient may have lost muscle from a fortuitously crucial place, but I suspect that increase in end-systolic cavity size was responsible, i.e. deterioration rather than improvement in left ventricular contractile ability. Although I believe passionately that the left ventricular end-diastolic pressure is very important it is only meaningful when it is considered in conjunction with the amount of work the ventricle is doing. If the end-diastolic pressure has fallen but the stroke volume has also fallen then this is not an improvement. The fall in end-diastolic pressure has to be associated with maintenance of the stroke work and nobody has yet shown that this occurs after operation. The other criterion of benefit would be that more of these patients are staying alive. Are they avoiding the development of atrial fibrillation and congestive failure in the very long term? Only time will show that.

*Barratt-Boyes:* It would be unhappy to let the previous remarks go completely unchallenged. What I haven't had demonstrated to my satisfaction is that in any individual patient with an obstructive type of this disease—and in our presentation we spoke only of that group—this obstruction necessarily disappears with time without first increasing in severity as a progressive phenomenon. Perhaps if we could relieve that obstruction at the appropriate time this progression might be slowed up, not necessarily prevented but appreciably altered. The abnormal mitral leaflet movement which we have demonstrated suggests to us that once this mitral leaflet assumes its abnormal shape this is a progressive phenomenon and the obstruction will gradually become more severe. The fact that it may in time disappear is not necessarily relevant to this argument. Maybe there are other factors which make it disappear, but I think we are jumping to conclusions to assume that we start at point A and end up at point C, and that the presence of obstruction at point B has nothing whatever to do with this progression. I feel that surgery does have a place in this disease, and maybe the timing of surgery is the thing which is of the greatest importance. Maybe it would be important to operate on these patients earlier rather than later, which is not what Dr Braunwald has suggested. I think this is entirely dependent on the mortality and morbidity of the operation and if this can be negligible I think a very good case can be made out for a relatively early surgical approach in patients with a significant gradient.

*Bentall:* What worries me is the dramatic success of some of the earlier operations which were really very limited myotomies. If they hadn't been quite so brilliant, and if some of my more recent operations in which I thought I had done a beautiful job, taking many grammes of muscle, had shown better results, I would be rather more impressed with myself than I am. I still believe that one should excise obstructing muscle. I may be wrong there, but I am not happy that we know yet completely what we are doing. I am sure we can forget our original concept of interfering with the mechanics of contraction. I believe that now we are mostly concerned with the removal of obstructing masses. This has a secondary beneficial effect, of course, on the degree of mitral incompetence, just as one relieves mitral incompetence very largely by the treatment of fixed aortic obstruction. There is one additional way in which the mitral valve can be incompetent early in systole. This systolic anterior movement could undoubtedly be due to involvement of papillary muscle in the disease.

This muscle is certainly part of the myocardium and is subject to exactly the same influences.

*Homan van der Heide:* My series was very limited and I can only say that in the only patient that we recatheterized there was an increase in cardiac output from 2·3 to 3·27 litres/min per square metre after operation, even when the patient was fibrillating. This is a definite improvement, and there was easier filling of the left ventricle, as shown on the apex cardiogram (Fig. 4, p. 168).

*Braunwald:* I think that the operative results are fully as good in idiopathic hypertrophic subaortic stenosis as they are in congenital valvular aortic stenosis or in acquired aortic stenosis. As for what is actually accomplished at operation, I think that any therapeutic manoeuvre that regularly takes patients out of Classes III–IV and puts them back to Class I or II, lowers the end-diastolic pressure, eliminates the gradient between the left ventricle and the aorta, does not lower the cardiac output, and does not lead to late myocardial deterioration and late deaths over a period up to ten years, is very acceptable indeed. That doesn't mean that the patients will remain well for 20 years but I doubt that patients with a prosthetic aortic valve will do better over such a long time span. I think that sufficient time has now elapsed to indicate that operation for IHSS is in the same range of effectiveness as is operation for the discrete obstructions to left ventricular outflow.

*Brock:* There has been much bandying about of the terms surgery and operation. This worries me a great deal because we are really talking mostly about operation as opposed to surgery. Again, it is suggested that it is a good surgical principle to excise or resect hypertrophied muscle. This I find very difficult to believe. I can understand it is sound surgery to do an incision by operation, but I am not satisfied that it is sound surgery to excise a lot of hypertrophied muscle by operation. I would give you that thought in regard to this question of the type of operation done on the outflow tract.

## REFERENCES

EPSTEIN, S. E. and MORROW, A. G. (1970) In *VI Wld Congr. Cardiology*, London.
LEV. M. and SIMPKINS, S. (1956) *Lab. Invest.* **5,** 396.
MALL, F. P. (1911) *Am. J. Anat.* **11, 211.**

Morrow, A. G., Lambrew, C. T. and Braunwald, E. (1964) In *Ciba Fdn Symp. Cardiomyopathies*, pp. 250–265. London: Churchill.

Shah, P. M. (1964) In *Ciba Fdn Symp. Cardiomyopathies*, pp. 26–27. London: Churchill.

Shah, P. M., Gramiak, R., Kramer, D. H. and Yu, P. N. (1968) *New Engl. J. Med.* **278,** 753.

# MORBID ANATOMY AND HISTOLOGY IN HYPERTROPHIC OBSTRUCTIVE CARDIOMYOPATHY

E. G. J. OLSEN

*Department of Pathology, Royal Postgraduate Medical School, Hammersmith Hospital, London*

SINCE the first full documentation by Teare (1958) of the pathological features of what is now referred to in England as hypertrophic obstructive cardiomyopathy (HOCM), no additional

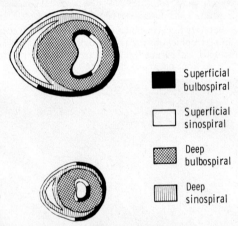

FIG. 1. Distribution of muscle bundles in the heart: diagrammatic representation of cross-sections, showing extreme hypertrophy of the septum. (After Wartman and Sounders, 1950.)

changes have been described. The typical asymmetry of the septal hypertrophy has been observed in most cases which have come to autopsy. The changes are best seen on cross-section of the heart, schematically represented in Fig. 1, where the anterior, lateral and posterior walls show moderate uniform hypertrophy of the myocardium. The extreme hypertrophy of the septum is striking. The muscle most frequently involved is the deep bulbospiral

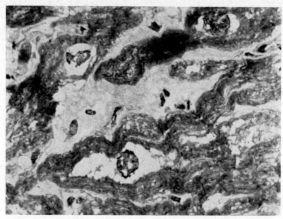

FIG. 2. Severely hypertrophied myocardial fibres in a patient with hypertrophic obstructive cardiomyopathy. Bizarre-shaped nuclei, and perinuclear haloes are clearly seen. (Frozen section; haematoxylin and eosin × 260.)

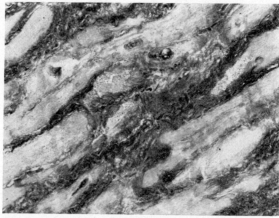

FIG. 3. Interruption of abnormal myocardial fibres by fibrous tissue. (Weigert's elastic-Van Gieson × 160.)

muscle with thinning or absence of the overlying superficial fasciculi. If the cardiac index is calculated, values of greater than unity are obtained (Menges, Brandenburg and Brown 1961). Although clinically the obstruction of the left ventricular outflow tract is capricious and may vary from day to day (Braunwald 1962), the changes observed pathologically explain the obstructive part of the condition. The septal hypertrophy usually extends to the aortic valve and may interfere with the normal function of the anterior leaflet of the mitral valve. No anatomical abnormality of the mitral valve has been observed in the cases we have studied.

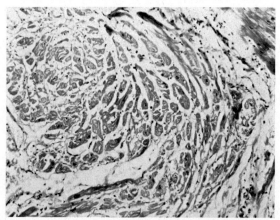

FIG. 4. A 'whorl' formation in a patient with hypertrophic obstructive cardiomyopathy. (Haematoxylin and eosin ×75.)

We studied material from ten cases at post-mortem, and biopsy tissue from 18 patients who underwent surgery. Histologically, disorientation of the myocardial fibres is present. Individually, they show extreme hypertrophy and values of up to 60 μm are not unusual in hypertrophic obstructive cardiomyopathy, whereas in left ventricular hypertrophy due to other causes fibres 20–25 μm wide (normal value 5–12 μm) are seen. Bizarre-shaped nuclei are observed within spaces referred to as nuclear haloes. These appearances are typical in this condition. The myocardial fibres adjacent to the perinuclear haloes have a 'moth-eaten' appearance (Fig. 2).

The presence of the endothelial-lined spaces described by Teare in 1958 and 1964 has been confirmed but these are not helpful in diagnosis. Interruption of the abnormal myocardial fibres by fibrous tissue is typical in these cases (Fig. 3). Serial sections of these areas show that fibrous tissue arises within the myocardial fibres and spreads towards the surface, replacing a variable amount of muscle tissue. This results in the observed shortening of the fibre and its termination in collagen tissue.

TABLE I

DETAILS OF PATIENTS USED AS CONTROLS AND NUMBER
OF THOSE WITH HOCM

| Clinical diagnosis | No. of patients | |
|---|---|---|
| Group I | | |
| Congestive cardiomyopathy | 4 | |
| Cardiomyopathy of unknown type | 4 | |
| Bacterial endocarditis | 1 | |
| Fallot's tetralogy | 4 | 38 |
| Ventricular septal defect | 2 | |
| Mitral stenosis | 3 | |
| Subaortic stenosis | 13 | |
| Aortic valve stenosis | 7 | |
| Group II | | |
| Hypertrophic obstructive cardiomyopathy | 18 | 18 |
| Total number of patients examined: | | 56 |

An additional point not previously described is the tendency of the myocardial bundles to form small 'whorls' and this, in our experience, is a fairly reliable histological guide to diagnosis (Fig. 4).

During the past three years we have concentrated on material obtained at operation, with particular emphasis on diagnostic reliability (Van Noorden, Olsen and Pearse 1970). In order to evaluate our observations on a numerical basis we have devised an index—the 'histological hypertrophic obstructive cardiomyopathy index' (H.H.I.), allotting points for each of the histological changes observed (fibrosis, bizarre nuclei, disappearing myocardial fibres with perinuclear spaces, whorls and short runs of fibres). This index was applied to the 18 patients who underwent surgery. Biopsy tissue, also obtained at operation, from 38 cases suffering from a variety of cardiac conditions served as controls.

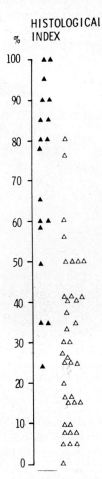

Each symbol represents one patient

▲ HOCM          △ NON-HOCM

FIG. 5. The histological index on which patients are plotted according to their percentage total score for the 5 typical histological characteristics of the myocardium in hypertrophic obstructive cardiomyopathy (HOCM).

These are tabulated in Table I. Each patient has been individually evaluated, and in Fig. 5 the scores are plotted as a percentage of the maximum possible. Some overlap occurs between the two groups and this emphasizes the fact that, in order to evaluate tissue

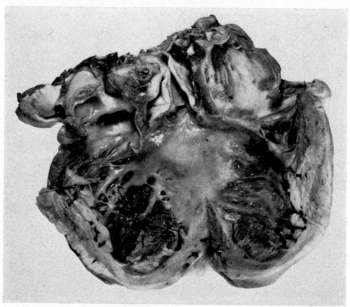

FIG. 6. The heart of a boy aged 7 years, showing dilatation of the left ventricular chamber and thrombus at the apex extending into the interventricular septum. The myocardial hypertrophy has been masked by the dilatation.

fully, ample material is needed to make a diagnosis: if only two or three histological features are seen, the positioning of the patient on the chart would be below the line where a reliable diagnosis is possible.

The description so far has been concerned with the 'classical' type of hypertrophic obstructive cardiomyopathy. There is, however, a group of patients who are difficult to classify clinically, who show little or no obstruction (Karatzas, Hamill and Sleight 1968). Five patients belonging to this group who were also difficult to categorize pathologically have so far been studied. Fig. 6 shows a heart from one of these patients, a boy aged seven years who presented with heart failure. A clinical diagnosis of 'cardiomyopathy' was made. This child also had two sisters, aged four and five years respectively, who both died of an identical cardiac condition. Fig. 7 shows a cross-section from the girl aged five years.*

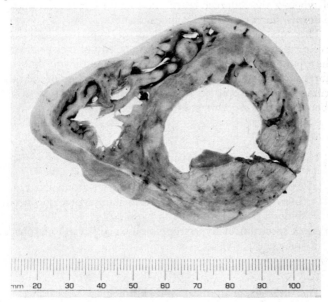

Fig. 7. Cross-section of a heart showing dilatation of the right and left ventricles. Myocardial hypertrophy is also present. From a girl aged 5 years.

Two hearts belonging to different, unrelated adults have also been examined. Dilatation of all chambers, endocardial thickening and occasional thrombus formation in the apical region are seen. Myocardial hypertrophy is present, but is not striking, being masked by the dilatation. This hypertrophy is uniform. The appearance differs, strikingly, from that in cases of hypertrophic obstructive cardiomyopathy.

Histologically, changes similar to those described in the 'classical' type are found, except that perinuclear haloes are not promi-

* The pathological material was sent to us by Drs Forrester and Watson from the Royal Manchester Children's Hospital.

nent but are present. Serial sections of two of the hearts have so far been examined. Whereas in the classical type abnormal fibres are aggregated in one area, usually but not always in the apex and septum, in these cases foci varying between 2 and 3 cm in diameter are scattered throughout the myocardium. The question arises of whether the different distribution of these scattered areas of abnormal fibres explains the clinical manifestations.

These studies suggest that a spectrum of 'hypertrophic obstructive cardiomyopathy' may exist. At one end of the spectrum is the typical asymmetric hypertrophy of the septum with abnormal fibres aggregated in one area, while at the other end of the spectrum no macroscopic changes are evident but foci of similar abnormal fibres are scattered through the myocardium.

## CONCLUSIONS

The following conclusions are drawn:
(1) A definite histological diagnosis is usually possible.
(2) Histology shows some overlap in the two groups examined.
(3) Distribution of areas with abnormal fibres precludes needle biopsy.
(4) A spectrum of hypertrophic obstructive cardiomyopathy may exist.

## SUMMARY

The morbid anatomical and histological appearances of hypertrophic obstructive cardiomyopathy (HOCM) have been examined in ten cases at post-mortem and in surgical material from 18 cases.

The diagnostic features have been described; 'whorl' formation was found to be of additional help in making a diagnosis.

Five cases who were difficult to classify clinically have also been studied. No morbid anatomical features of hypertrophic obstructive cardiomyopathy were found. Histologically, small aggregates of abnormal myocardial fibres identical to those of HOCM were scattered throughout the myocardium, whereas in the classical form they were found in only one large aggregate at the apex and interventricular septum.

It is suggested that a spectrum of hypertrophic obstructive cardiomyopathy may exist.

## REFERENCES

BRAUNWALD, E. (1962) *Circulation* **26,** 161.

KARATZAS, N. B., HAMILL, J. and SLEIGHT, P. (1968) *Br. Heart J.* **30,** 826.

MENGES, H. J., BRANDENBURG, R. O. and BROWN, A. L. (1961) *Circulation*
    **24,** 1126.

TEARE, R. D. (1958) *Br. Heart J.* **20,** 1.

TEARE, R. D. (1964) In *Ciba Fdn Symp. Cardiomyopathies*, p. 11. London:
    Churchill.

VAN NOORDEN, S., OLSEN, E. G. J. and PEARSE, A. G. E. (1970) *Cardiovasc.*
    *Res.* in press.

WARTMAN, W. B. and SOUNDERS, J. C. (1950) *Archs Path.* **50,** 329–346.

# HISTOCHEMISTRY AND ELECTRON MICROSCOPY OF THE HEART IN HYPERTROPHIC OBSTRUCTIVE CARDIOMYOPATHY

SUSAN VAN NOORDEN AND A. G. E. PEARSE

*Department of Histochemistry, Royal Postgraduate Medical School, Hammersmith Hospital, London*

AT the 1964 Ciba Foundation Symposium on cardiomyopathies one of us presented a paper on the histochemistry and electron microscopy of the heart in five cases of hypertrophic obstructive cardiomyopathy (HOCM) compared with two controls (Pearse 1964). We have now studied 54 patients consisting of 16 HOCM cases and 38 controls, including the original series which has been re-assessed (Table I).

### TABLE I

PATIENT MATERIAL

| Clinical diagnosis | | No. of patients |
|---|---|---|
| Hypertrophic obstructive cardiomyopathy | | 16 |
| Congestive cardiomyopathy | 4 | |
| Cardiomyopathy of unknown type | 4 | |
| Bacterial endocarditis | 1 | |
| Fallot's tetralogy | 4 | 38 |
| Ventricular septal defect | 2 | |
| Mitral stenosis | 3 | |
| Subaortic stenosis | 13 | |
| Aortic valve stenosis | 7 | |

### MATERIAL

Samples of muscle from the obstructed area of the left ventricular outflow tract were taken from cases of HOCM and control samples were usually from a similar area in cases of subaortic stenosis, mitral stenosis, etc. Small pieces of muscle from the apex were occasionally supplied in addition.

### METHODS

When the tissue sample was large enough it was divided into four parts, which were treated as follows:

(1) For investigations on fresh-frozen cryostat sections the tissue was frozen in Arcton 22, pre-cooled in liquid nitrogen to $-158\ °C$;

(2) For study of the formaldehyde-induced fluorescence of catecholamines the tissue was frozen as above, then dried in a thermoelectric freeze-dryer, exposed to formaldehyde vapour at 60 °C and embedded in wax (Falck *et al.* 1962);

(3) For electron microscopy the tissue was chopped into 1 mm cubes, fixed in osmium tetroxide or glutaraldehyde, dehydrated through alcohols and embedded in Epon;

(4) For further histochemical investigations on pre-fixed frozen sections or routine paraffin embedding the tissue was fixed in cold formol calcium for 24 hours and then stored until required in gum sucrose at 4 °C.

## Staining

Histochemical staining was carried out on cryostat sections as shown in Table II. Unless otherwise stated the methods used were those cited by Pearse (1960).

Thin sections for electron microscopy were stained with lead citrate and uranyl acetate.

### RESULTS

As with the histology, the histochemical and ultrastructural findings were the same in the apex and the outflow tract. This confirms the conclusions of Cohen and co-workers (1964), McCallister and Brown (1967) and Meessen (1968).

## Histochemistry

In the HOCM cases histochemical techniques usually revealed the same pattern of enzyme activity and increase in the number of cellular organelles that was shown by Pearse (1964). There were usually patchy increases in the number of mitochondria, shown by the activity of their dehydrogenases (Figs. 1 and 2), and increased numbers of lysosomes, shown by the acid phosphatase and non-specific esterase (Figs. 3 and 4) they contained. However the control cases with ordinary hypertrophy often showed the same type of enzyme distribution and increased activity as the HOCM cases and in some of the HOCM cases no marked increase could be seen.

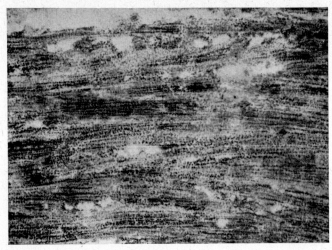

FIG. 1. Succinate dehydrogenase reaction showing normal
distribution of mitochondria. (× 402.)

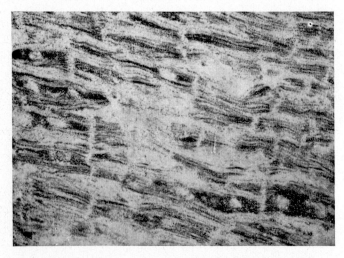

FIG. 2. Succinate dehydrogenase reaction showing patchy
increases in mitochondria (mitochondriosis) in a case of
HOCM. (× 402.)

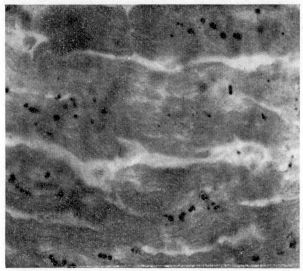

Fig. 3.  Non-specific esterase (α-naphthyl) reaction showing
normal lysosomal reaction.  (× 452.)

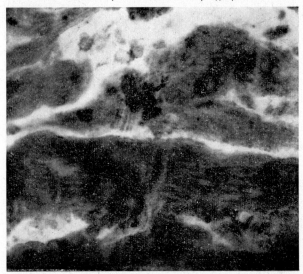

Fig. 4.  Non-specific esterase (α-naphthyl) reaction showing
increased number of lysosomes in cardiomyopathy.  (× 452.)

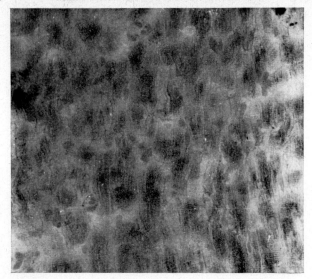

FIG. 5. Normal distribution of glycogen. PAS reaction.
(×452.)

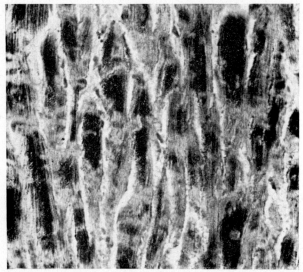

FIG. 6. Glycogen in a case of HOCM showing perinuclear
'pooling'. PAS reaction. (×452.)

Myosin ATPase was evenly distributed in the muscle fibres of both HOCM and control hearts wherever the muscle fibres were intact, and no difference was noted in the size and distribution of the blood vessels. Cholinesterase was absent except in occasional

## TABLE II

### HISTOCHEMICAL TECHNIQUES

| *Substance shown* | *Method* |
| --- | --- |
| Glycogen | Periodic acid/Schiff (diastase-digested control) |
| Neutral fat | Oil Red O |
| Lipofuscin | Schmorl |
| Dehydrogenases | Monotetrazolium–cobalt |
|   Reduced nicotinamide adenine dinucleotide dehydrogenase (NADH-D) | |
|   Reduced nicotinamide adenine dinucleotide phosphate dehydrogenase (NADPH-D) | |
| Succinate dehydrogenase | |
| Lactate dehydrogenase | |
|   Isocitrate dehydrogenase | |
|   β-hydroxybutyrate dehydrogenase | |
| Oxidases | |
|   Monoamine oxidase | Glenner |
|   Cytochrome oxidase | Burstone |
| Lysosomal hydrolases | |
|   Acid phosphatase | Barka and Anderson (1963) |
|   Non-specific esterase | |
|     indoxyl | Holt |
|     α-naphthyl | Barka and Anderson (1963) |
| Cholinesterase | Gomori |
| Alkaline phosphatase | Burstone |
| Adenosine triphosphatase | Padykula and Herman |
| Phosphorylase | Eränkö and Paklama (1961) |
| Glycogen synthetase | Takeuchi and Glenner (1961) |
| 'Leucine aminopeptidase' (metal-dependent aminopeptidase) | Nachlas, Crawford and Seligman |

nerves and conducting system cells (one control case only). 'Leucine aminopeptidase' (metal-dependent aminopeptidase) was absent except in occasional mast cells and macrophages.

Fat droplets were rarely found in the HOCM muscle but were occasionally seen in controls. Lipofuscin pigment granules were

HISTOCHEMISTRY

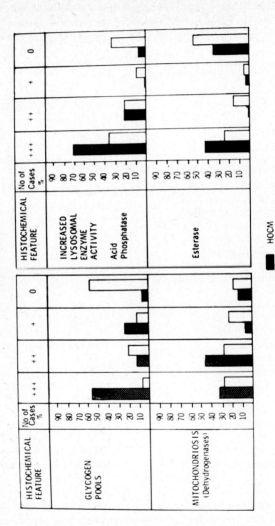

Fig. 7.  Chart of histochemical results.

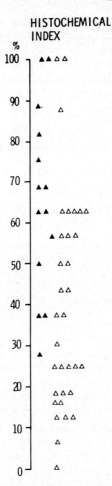

## HISTOCHEMICAL INDEX

Each symbol represents one patient

▲ HOCM          △ NON-HOCM

FIG. 8. Histochemical index for 14 HOCM and 33 non-HOCM cases.

commonly present in more than normal numbers in both HOCM muscle and controls.

In the HOCM muscle, as previously described by Pearse (1964), accumulations of glycogen could often be seen around the nuclei in the affected areas (Figs. 5 and 6) and although glycogen levels were quite high in both HOCM and control muscle this 'pooling' distribution was fairly typical of the HOCM hearts, though not confined to them. Table III describes the incidence and degree of glycogen pooling among our samples.

TABLE III

INCIDENCE AND DEGREE OF GLYCOGEN POOLING

| Glycogen pools | HOCM | | Non-HOCM (excluding congestives) | |
|---|---|---|---|---|
| | No. of patients | % of total | No. of patients | % of total |
| 3+ | 9 | 56·2 | 3 | 8·8 |
| 2+ | 2 | 12·5 | 7 | 20·7 |
| 1+ | 4 | 25 | 4 | 11·7 |
| 0 | 1 | 6·3 | 20 | 58·8 |
| Total cases | 16 | | 34 | |

Two enzymes concerned with glycogen metabolism, glycogen synthetase (uridine diphosphate glucose glycogen transferase) and phosphorylase, did not show any difference in activity between HOCM muscles and controls. Glycogen pooling remains the most useful though not infallible distinguishing histochemical characteristic of HOCM muscle.

A histochemical index was prepared for each case in the same way as described for the histology (Olsen 1971). The following four characteristics were assessed on an arbitrary scale from 0 to 3+ : glycogen pooling, mitochondriosis, increased level of acid-phosphatase activity, increased level of non-specific esterase activity. It can be seen (Figs. 7 and 8) that the area of overlap is too great for this to be a useful aid to diagnosis of HOCM as opposed to cardiac hypertrophy due to other causes.

On the basis of silver staining and the formaldehyde-induced fluorescence of noradrenaline it was suggested (Pearse 1964) that the number of sympathetic nerves and the amount of noradrenaline was increased in the HOCM muscle compared with the

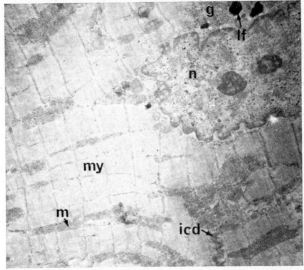

Fig. 9. Electron micrograph. Subaortic stenosis. n=nucleus, g=glycogen, m=mitochondria, my=myofibril, icd= intercalated disc, lf=lipofuscin granule. (×4500.)

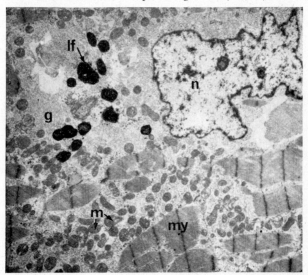

Fig. 10. Electron micrograph. HOCM. Labelling as for Fig. 9. Note accumulation of glycogen and disruption of myofibrils. (×4500.)

controls. This hypothesis has not been confirmed. We have found that connective tissue autofluorescence with a similar emission spectrum to that of noradrenaline (485 nm) tends to confuse the picture considerably. Because of the fibrosis which is such a prominent feature of the HOCM muscle there was often more fluorescence than in the controls but no definite increase in nerves or noradrenaline could be seen by this method or with the ethyl-amine-silver oxalate stain.

*Electron microscopy*

In several cases the electron microscopy corresponded with Pearse's (1964) description. The most striking feature of severely affected myocardium was the 'dystrophic' appearance of the muscle with disappearing myofibrils and occasionally complete disintegration of fibres. Frequently mitochondria were present in greater than normal numbers round the nuclei and usually their structure was normal though sometimes they were damaged with swollen and disrupted cristae. In many cases accumulations of glycogen granules could be seen. Intercalated discs did not show any consistent abnormality. The sarcotubular system was often distended and the muscle appeared vacuolated (Figs. 9 and 10).

The damaged areas were very patchily distributed and because of the sampling error due to the small size of the electron micro-scopy tissue blocks it was possible to find sections composed entirely of muscle which looked quite normal apart from its hypertrophy.

In general the ultrastructure of the muscle confirmed the histological findings. The control muscle was usually less damaged than the HOCM muscle but where abnormalities were seen they were of the same type as in the HOCM cases. It was possible to find disrupted fibres, contraction banding, mitochondrial aggre-gates, etc.

An ultrastructural index on the same lines as the histological and histochemical indices already described showed an even greater area of overlap.

DISCUSSION

Histochemical studies have shown that the enzyme activity of the HOCM hearts for all the systems studied was normal or slightly higher than normal—at least, *in vitro* when supplied with the appropriate substrates—and no difference was observed between the HOCM hearts and the hypertrophied control muscle. Where the muscle fibres were damaged a disturbance in the distribution of the enzyme stain was apparent but the type of damage was the same in both.

Meerson (1969) has postulated three stages in compensatory cardiac hypertrophy. The first follows the initial state of damage with no hypertrophy but an increase in energy production and protein synthesis which reduces the concentration of muscle glycogen.

The second stage is that of relatively stable hyperfunction in which hypertrophy leads to restoration of normal levels of glycogen and activity of the muscle.

The third stage is reached when the load falling on the heart exceeds its capacity for performing work and myocardial insufficiency results.

These stages have been produced in rats by Vihert and Pozdyunina (1969) and their results on enzyme staining in the second stage correspond in most respects with ours in these diseased human hearts. We suggest that the biopsies we have studied come from hearts in the second stage of relatively stable hyperfunction and hypertrophy.

Wartman (1969) has pointed out that the heart can react to injury in only a few ways (inflammation, hypertrophy, degeneration, necrosis and fibrosis) and it is consistent with this concept that we can show no specific difference between the heart muscle from HOCM and from hypertrophy of a more usual aetiology.

A high level of glycogen was found by Meessen and Poche (1967) in their ultrastructural study of idiopathic hypertrophic subaortic stenosis and an increased glycogen content was found biochemically in the heart muscle of rats stressed by running in a treadmill (Drasnin et al. 1958). Other biochemical evidence is for a preliminary decrease in glycogen content of hypertrophied heart muscle followed by a return to normality (Badeer 1968), but a patchy increase such as we have found might be concealed in a biochemical study.

Two groups of workers have recently examined myocardium from HOCM cases at the electron microscope level and have found the same type of damage as we have described here (Meessen and Poche 1967; Snijder, De Jong and Meijer 1970). Leyton and Sonnenblick's (1969) findings in hypertrophied hearts also correspond with these and their work underlines the non-specific nature of the lesions we encounter.

Thus we conclude that up to now histochemical and ultrastructural studies of the myocardium in cases of HOCM reveal only non-specific changes due to the extreme hypertrophy of the muscle, and no specific defect has been found which could be used as an infallible diagnostic criterion in this clinically well-defined disease.

### SUMMARY

Myocardial biopsies from 16 cases of HOCM and 38 cases of cardiac hypertrophy due to other causes were examined by histochemical and electron microscopical techniques. The results added confirmation to the histological studies but no lesion specific to HOCM was found.

## REFERENCES

BADEER, H. S. (1968) Prog. cardiovasc. Dis. **11,** 53–63.

BARKA, T. and ANDERSON, P. J. (1963) Histochemistry: Theory, Practise and Bibliography. New York: Harper and Row.

COHEN, J., EFFAT, H., GOODWIN, J. E., OAKLEY, C. M. and STEINER, R. E. (1964) Br. Heart J. **26,** 16–32.

DRASNIN, R., HUGHES, J. T., KRAUSE, R. F. and VAN LIERE, E. J. (1958) Proc. Soc. exp. Biol. Med. **99,** 438–439.

ERÄNKÖ, O. and PAKLAMA, A. (1961) J. Histochem. Cytochem. **9,** 585.

FALCK, B., HILLARP, N. Å., THIEME, G. and TORP, A. (1962) J. Histochem. Cytochem. **10,** 348–354.

LEYTON, R. A. and SONNENBLICK, E. H. (1969) Am. J. med. Sci. **258,** 304–327.

McCALLISTER, B. D. and BROWN, A. L. (1967) Am. J. Cardiol. **19,** 142.

MEERSON, F. Z. (1969) Circulation Res. **25,** Suppl. II.

MEESSEN, H. (1968) Am. J. Cardiol. **22,** 319–327.

MEESSEN, H. and POCHE, R. (1967) Anglo-Ger. Med. Rev. **4,** 73–87.

OLSEN, E. G. J. (1971) This volume, pp. 183–191.

PEARSE, A. G. E. (1960) Histochemistry, Theoretical and Applied, 2nd ed. London: Churchill.

PEARSE, A. G. E. (1964) In Ciba Fdn Symp. Cardiomyopathies, pp. 132–164. London: Churchill.

SNIJDER, J., DE JONG, J. and MEIJER, A. E. F. H. (1970) J. Path. Bact. **100,** Pi.

TAKEUCHI, T. and GLENNER, G. G. (1961) J. Histochem. Cytochem. **9,** 304–316.

VIHERT, A. M. and POZDYUNINA, N. H. (1969) Virchows Arch. path. Anat. Physiol. **347,** 44–56.

WARTMAN, W. B. (1969) Ann. N.Y. Acad. Sci. **156,** 7–13.

# DISCUSSION

*Silver:* When you say you found no abnormality of the mitral valve do you mean an abnormality in the sense used by Björk, Hulquist and Lodin (1961), Dr Olsen?

*Olsen:* Yes.

*Silver:* Were glycogen stains done on material from the three children who showed little or no obstruction?

*Olsen:* Yes, and increased glycogen was present but was not as prevalent as in the classical type.

*Silver:* Do the small granules you called glycogen show any differential staining with lead or uranyl acetate?

*Van Noorden:* Staining with aqueous uranyl acetate showed that some of the smaller particles in these pools at the electron microscope level may be ribonucleoprotein (Revel 1964) but the vast majority are identified as glycogen granules.

*Nellen:* Some of the macroscopic cross-sections from your cases, Dr Olsen, looked very much like those described by Bernheim (1910). Could some of his cases have been examples of obstructive cardiomyopathy?

*Olsen:* I cannot answer this with certainty, not having seen these cases, but some of our patients did not show severe asymmetric hypertrophy.

*Nellen:* Perhaps the obstruction in the right ventricle is purely a bulge from the left into the right ventricle, so the right ventricular obstruction could really be a Bernheim effect?

*Olsen:* Yes.

*Emanuel:* Dr Olsen, your concept of a histological spectrum is most attractive. I believe you have examined a few cases with mild fixed aortic valve obstruction in which there was left ventricular hypertrophy quite out of keeping with the degree of valve obstruction. What were your findings in this small group?

*Olsen:* The light microscopy findings showed hypertrophic changes only and none of the features I have described in the two groups of hypertrophic obstructive cardiomyopathy.

*Braunwald:* In 1964 we were measuring noradrenaline histochemically in cardiac tissue of a variety of patients and after seeing Dr Pearse's material at the meeting here (Pearse 1964) we took biopsies from 13 patients, seven of whom had IHSS. As an arbitrary control Drs Sonnenblick, Morrow and I used biopsy

material from the right ventricular outflow tract of six patients
with Fallot's tetralogy. There was a marked decrease in noradrenaline concentration in the resected tissue of patients with IHSS.
These results certainly did not support the concept of a hyper-
sympathetic condition. It is interesting to see that your further
studies also do not confirm this concept which was presented in
1964.

*Goodwin:* Were the patients with IHSS those who had reached
the congestive state? In other words could they have depleted
their noradrenaline? I imagine that doesn't happen with Fallot's
tetralogy because except in infants and much older groups
congestive heart failure doesn't usually occur.

*Braunwald:* Only one was in a congestive state.

*Silver:* The clinicians have spoken here about a progression in
patients with HOCM. We have seen biopsies taken at ventriculomyotomy in such patients, then examined their hearts at autopsies
five or six years later and noticed changes in the histology of the
muscle that, in our view, suggested a progression of the changes.
To test this we examined the seven sectioned hearts I referred to
earlier (p. 177) and found that the histological changes could be
divided into four classes. In the first, large bizarre muscle fibres
like those Dr Olsen has just described were present in the centre
of the left ventricular wall but there was very little interstitial
fibrous tissue. In the second, the bizarre fibres were larger and
the pattern more florid, while the amount of interstitial tissue was
increased. In the third, a progressive increase in connective tissue
was clearly seen surrounding the bizarre fibres and separating their
truncated ends. In the fourth, the few bizarre fibres that remained
looked like islands in a sea of connective tissue. This fibrosis was
confined to the central left ventricular wall and was not difficult
to differentiate from the pattern of fibrosis that occurs in patients
with ischaemic heart disease. In both the third and fourth classes
degenerating muscle fibres surrounded by small collections of
macrophages and lymphocytes could be seen. These collections of
mononuclear cells are not evidence of a myocarditis; rather, they
represent the removal of degenerating fibres. Histological changes
corresponding to the four classes described above could be found
in small areas in individual hearts but overall the changes of one
class seem to predominate in a heart. We then tried to see whether
a relationship existed between the four classes of change and the

duration of the patient's illness, defined as "between the time symptoms were first noted, or a heart murmur was found, and the time of death". Our statistician found a trend that suggested such an association. Thus, although we cannot say with certainty that the histological changes are progressive, there is a suggestion that they are.

I agree with Dr Olsen that needle biopsy is not of much use in the diagnosis of HOCM. As I mentioned, tiny focal areas showing a bizarre muscle pattern like that seen in Class I or Class II may be seen in hearts hypertrophied as a result of conditions other than HOCM. If a needle biopsy passed through such an area a pathologist would have tremendous difficulty deciding whether or not the patient had HOCM. Thus, to establish a diagnosis with certainty a full thickness left ventricular section is needed to see whether the bizarre muscle pattern is present in the central area of the left ventricular wall.

*Olsen:* We have observed all the stages of severity you have described in our surgical material—irrespective of the length of history—with little or no change when the patient came to postmortem. On the other hand we have seen patients who died without previous surgery who only showed mild histological changes even with relatively long histories. It is possible that surgery itself may have induced fibrosis (your fourth stage). Therefore, in our experience we cannot be certain that progression takes place.

One point of clarification: did you suggest that fibrosis seen in hypertrophic obstructive cardiomyopathy is similar or dissimilar to myocardial infarction? I think it is the remaining myocardial fibre which makes distinction possible. The isolated fibre in myocardial infarction shows none of the histological features I have described in hypertrophic obstructive cardiomyopathy. In none of your slides did you show any particular nuclear abnormalities or any perinuclear halos.

*Silver:* The fibrosis one sees in what I call Class IV cannot be equated in any way with the type of fibrosis one sees in ischaemic heart disease. The muscle fibres remaining at this stage are certainly quite bizarre.

*Burchell:* A problem touched on in 1964 was the relationship of phaeochromocytoma and adrenaline in myocarditis. I believe that the lesions in phaeochromocytoma were dissimilar to those reported in idiopathic hypertrophy (see Wolstenholme and O'Connor 1964). Dr Olsen, have you studied these cases again to see whether there are any similarities between the isolated areas of the muscle where the fibrosis has occurred?

*Olsen:* We have not gone into this in any great detail, and we have studied only one case since 1964 with phaeochromocytoma. This showed 'ordinary' hypertrophy and fibrosis of the myocardium. I agree with you that the changes were dissimilar.

*Wigle:* The group here in London have rather gone out of their way to express their viewpoint that the obstruction may be incidental in this condition. Our view has always been that this is a primary myocardial disease which may be progressive. When we have spoken to such patients about having cardiac surgery, or when we published articles on the results of surgery, we have suggested that we are not affecting the primary myocardial disease but rather are operating to relieve the outflow tract obstruction. We submit that the operation is palliative, but it is highly palliative and highly effective in the relief of symptoms, the relief of the outflow tract obstruction, the lowering of the end-diastolic pressure and the abolition of the mitral regurgitation. We would submit that the fact that patients with increasing obstruction and worsening symptomatology often develop left atrial and ventricular hypertrophy preoperatively, and show regression of this hypertrophy postoperatively, is evidence that the outflow tract obstruction was indeed having a deleterious effect. Left ventricular ejection time is also shortened by successful surgery, and if the length of systole is one of the determinants of myocardial oxygen consumption we would submit that this is also a beneficial effect. On the basis of these and other considerations we believe that it is worth offering surgery to these patients when there is evidence that the outflow tract obstruction is important. But there are two parts to the disease, and we would not claim that relieving the outflow tract obstruction stops the progression of the underlying myocardial process, if such occurs. From our own observations and Dr Silver's pathological observations in our own cases, the obstruction to outflow is not incidental, but is one important facet of the condition, so if we can deal with it adequately and effectively we should do so.

*Olsen:* The patients in the second group I described do not have an outflow tract obstruction. They may present first with congestion and are therefore difficult to classify. Have you seen such a patient in your pathological material?

*Silver:* No, but aren't most of these cases children?

*Olsen:* No; we studied two hearts from adults who were not related to the three children in that group nor were they related to one another.

*Wigle:* Your second group of cases looked like congestive cardiomyopathy with a dilated ventricle. One of the seven cases that Dr Silver sectioned serially was clinically a hypertrophic cardiomyopathy without obstruction, verified angiographically and by pressure tracings, and this patient had the same type of myocardial defect as did the patients with outflow obstruction. In other words patients can have the same myocardial defect and either have obstruction or no obstruction.

*Olsen:* But these belong to the group where the abnormal fibres are in one continuous band and are not haphazardly distributed.

*Wigle:* Correct.

*Hallidie-Smith:* Do these cases who present for the first time in the congestive phase have the same histology as our patients whom we have watched pass from the obstructive to the congestive stage?

*Olsen:* Yes, but it is a matter of distribution. Those who had obstruction first and went into the congestive phase may not show asymmetric hypertrophy but they still show abnormal fibres in one continuous band (usually extending from the apex to the aortic valve). The others, who present with congestion in the first instance, show these abnormal fibres scattered throughout the whole of the left ventricular myocardium, in small discontinuous aggregates 2 to 3 cm in diameter.

*Silver:* Does this finding upset the lumpers?

*Oakley:* Not at all! The distribution of the dystrophic cells may well vary from case to case. Whatever you feel about the possible heterogeneity of the disease it seems that a basic improvement in function can be achieved by the use of practolol. We haven't yet had a chance to see what it does in long-term oral treatment, but it is a very exciting new development that we shall watch with great interest, particularly now that we have echocardiograms to provide objective evidence on serial study.

*Goodwin:* On the question of surgery I am about mid-way

between Dr Wigle and Dr Oakley. The evidence we have seen here suggests that surgery still has a place and that there are patients who can be improved by surgical treatment. But I don't think this means that outflow tract obstruction is necessarily any more than an incident in the disease. Hammersmith is not entirely anti-surgery!

*Olsen:* I examined patients diagnosed as having congestive cardiomyopathy but who showed a non-specific picture histologically and no abnormal fibres.

*Goodwin:* I am sure that fundamentally there are indeed two different main groups of cardiomyopathies: the *congestive* type with the *large cavity* but not much hypertrophy, and by contrast, the type with much *hypertrophy* and a *small cavity* that we have been discussing and which we call HOCM or IHSS. The possibility of an overlap or spectrum of such diseases, as you said, of course cannot be denied.

## REFERENCES

BERNHEIM, E. (1910) *Revue Méd.* **30,** 785.

BJÖRK, V. O., HULQUIST, G. and LODIN, H. (1961) *J. thorac. cardiovasc. Surg.* **41,** 659.

PEARSE, A. G. E. (1964) In *Ciba Fdn Symp. Cardiomyopathies,* p. 132. London: Churchill.

REVEL, J. P. (1964) *J. Histochem. Cytochem.* **12,** 104–113.

WOLSTENHOLME, G. E. W. and O'CONNOR, M. (eds.) (1964) In *Ciba Fdn Symp. Cardiomyopathies,* p. 313. London: Churchill.

# SUMMING UP

## Dr E. Braunwald

ALTHOUGH we have had presented to us an enormous amount of valuable descriptive material concerning hypertrophic subaortic stenosis and although many issues have been clarified, we do not appear to be any closer to an understanding of the fundamental defect in this disease than we were at the Ciba Foundation Symposium in 1964. Moreover, I do not readily see, coming out of this meeting, any obvious directions that we can take to increase our comprehension of the underlying abnormality responsible for the clinical, pathological and haemodynamic changes characteristic of these conditions.

So much for the negative side of the coin. What have we learned in a positive sense since our last meeting in 1964? A basic question that many of us asked six years ago was whether obstruction ever precedes hypertrophy in idiopathic hypertrophic subaortic stenosis (IHSS). The experiences of the past few years and, in particular, the histological data presented at this meeting indicate that hypertrophy always precedes obstruction and that the obstruction may actually be incidental. In many patients, obviously, this is an extremely important incident.

Six years ago many of us felt very proud if we were able to establish the diagnosis of IHSS clinically and then have it confirmed in the laboratory, but we are now in a situation in which it is really inexcusable to miss the diagnosis from clinical examination.

The genetic transmission is becoming clearer, as Dr Emanuel has pointed out, at least from a descriptive point of view. The fact that there are two distinct presentations of the disease—familial and sporadic—is worth following up in depth. The history of medicine is replete with examples of diseases in which the clues for the underlying illness came from the observation that in some instances there was a familial association.

The question of whether there is obstruction or whether the gradient can be explained on the basis of catheter trapping has, as Dr Wigle pointed out, been pretty much resolved. The reason why there was so much turmoil in the U.S.A. about this in 1965 and 1966 was that many of us were then beginning to advise operative correction in a significant number of patients. Our operative follow-ups were on a relatively small number of patients and when Dr Criley presented his work we were dreadfully afraid that perhaps these operations had been for nothing. It has now become clear, I think, that it is not difficult to recognize catheter entrapment; actually it had not been a problem to those of us who were studying these patients routinely by means of trans-septal rather than retrograde left ventricular catheterization. The intraventricular pressure gradient resulting from catheter entrapment occurs more frequently in hypertrophied than normal hearts and it is particularly common in IHSS. Dr Criley did not visualize the obstruction on his cineangiograms because most of his studies were carried out, I believe, in the right anterior oblique projection, a projection in which it is almost impossible to see the obstruction, even when it can be readily observed in other projections.

We have learned a great deal about the contribution of the mitral valve to the obstruction in the last six years. The observations presented by Drs Wigle, Barratt-Boyes, Shah and Oakley here, and studies by Drs Ross and Simon, indicate that the mitral valve forms at least a portion of the boundary of the area of obstruction. Professor Björk considered that it constituted a very major component of the obstruction and perhaps it does in a very small number of patients. But I think it is clear that it forms at least 90° and perhaps 180° of the total obstructing circumference in most patients with IHSS. This has been a step forward.

The fact that we haven't heard anything about hypertension or the hyperkinetic heart syndrome here suggests that neither are likely to be important links in the condition that we are discussing. Enough people with an intense interest in this condition have been looking out for these associations, and it seems that if they exist they do so on a chance basis. That is, any associations of IHSS with hypertension or the hyperkinetic heart syndrome are coincidental, not causal.

There has been substantial progress in the understanding of the natural history of the disease. Although the course varies enormously among different patients, with a few ups and downs the course is mostly downhill, over a fairly long period of time. I think Dr Oakley and Professor Goodwin have made a helpful contribution by emphasizing that loss of obstruction can take place in patients as they deteriorate clinically. On the other hand, it has also been shown today that exactly the reverse can take place.

I would not venture to comment on the use of practolol at this very early stage but, as Dr Kristinsson and Professor Goodwin have pointed out, beta-blockade with pronethalol and propranolol has been disappointing. Six years ago when some of us presented the initial work with acute blockade and the earliest studies with oral treatment, we all had more hope for antiadrenergic therapy in this condition. Now it seems that few seriously symptomatic patients can be spared operative treatment by β-adrenergic blockade, although perhaps operation may be delayed for a while in patients with obstruction. It will be interesting to see whether practolol turns out to be different from propranolol.

While medical treatment has been somewhat disappointing, surgical treatment has been enormously and surprisingly gratifying to many. I took the position in 1962 (Braunwald, Brockenbrough and Morrow 1962) that we were dealing with a cardiomyopathy and that the most one could possibly accomplish with surgical treatment was to convert a patient with an obstructive cardiomyopathy to a patient with a non-obstructive cardiomyopathy. Mr Barratt-Boyes, Drs Bigelow and Wigle, Dr Morrow, Dr Kirklin and others have all had very gratifying results in the past six years. There is also relief of mitral regurgitation with operation in most instances.

I don't think that there is really any polarization of views about the classification of the disease. Lord Brock first pointed out this condition in the context of obstruction to left ventricular outflow. The major lesions which produce obstruction to left ventricular outflow include supravalvular aortic stenosis (familial, sporadic, with or without mental retardation, and having various anatomical loci). In valvular aortic stenosis we have the congenital type with its various subgroups, and the acquired type. In subvalvular aortic stenosis we recognize at least three groups: the congenital membranous, the secondary hypertrophic group of which Lord Brock has reminded us again (p. 47), and finally the muscular hypertrophic type, i.e. IHSS or HOCM. In this latter group there are both familial and sporadic types.

In one sense we are all blind men trying to describe an elephant.

Those blind men who are surgeons consider IHSS to be a form of obstruction to left ventricular outflow. On the other hand, those blind men who are physicians classify this disease primarily as a cardiomyopathy. I like the Goodwin (1970) classification of cardio-myopathies: (1) *congestive*—and in this group we recognize the familial and non-familial types; (2) *restrictive*, a smaller group; (3) *obliterative;* and (4) *hypertrophic* with or without obstruction. This category may also be familial in some instances.

TABLE I

| OBSTRUCTION TO LEFT VENTRICULAR OUTFLOW | CARDIOMYOPATHIES |
|---|---|
| I *Supravalvular* | I *Congestive* |
|   (A) Familial |   (A) Familial |
|   (B) Non-familial |   (B) Non-familial |
|     (1) With mental retardation | II *Restrictive* |
|     (2) Without mental retardation | III *Obliterative* |
| II *Valvular* | |
|   (A) Congenital | |
|   (B) Acquired | |
| III *Subaortic* | IV *Hypertrophic* |
|   (A) Congenital membranous (or fibrous) |   (A) Without obstruction to left ventricular outflow |
|   (B) Secondary hypertrophic | |
|   (C) Idiopathic hypertrophic = |   (B) With obstruction to left ventricular outflow |
|     (1) Familial |     (1) Familial |
|     (2) Non-familial |     (2) Non-familial |

Table I describes these two approaches to classification. (Note that IIIC under *Obstruction to left ventricular outflow* is identical to category IVB under *Cardiomyopathies*.) It is important that in the future we define the population that we describe as specifically as possible. I don't think it matters much whether we use IHSS or HOCM as designations, but it is very important to define our patient population because there has been some ambiguity in the literature and even a little ambiguity in the discussion here. Some people just include patients with documented obstruction to left ventricular outflow and these might be the purest, most restrictive group. Some, like myself, include among patients with

IHSS those patients with left ventricular hypertrophy who are first-degree relatives of patients with IHSS and obstruction. A third group of clinicians are least restrictive and will include any patient with left ventricular hypertrophy, regardless of the presence or absence of obstruction, or familial association. Because of these widely differing approaches, careful definition is of considerable importance.

## REFERENCES

BRAUNWALD, E., BROCKENBROUGH, E. C. and MORROW, A. G. (1962) *Circulation* **26,** 161.
GOODWIN, J, F. (1970) *Lancet* **1**, 731–739.

# SUBJECT INDEX*

*Printed by William Clowes & Sons Limited, London, Colchester and Beccles*